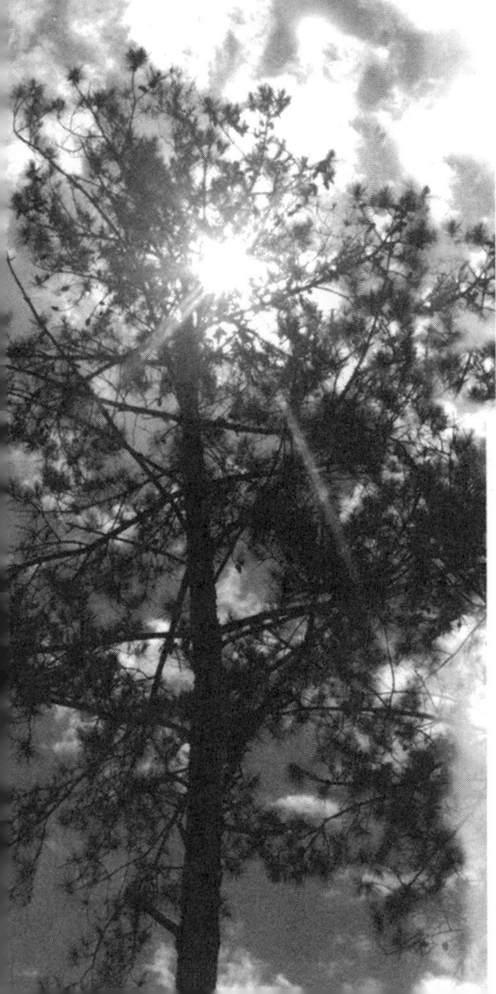

"There is no death, only a change of worlds."

—Chief Seattle

*This book is dedicated to Bill Waxman
and George D'Arbanville, our Dads,
whose laughter, love and memories
helped guide our journey.*

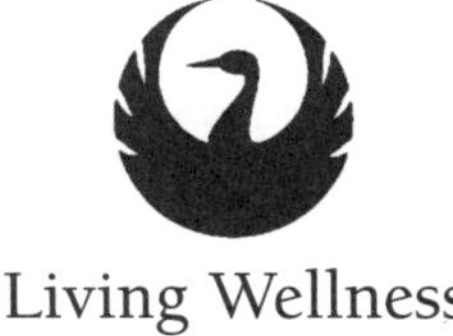

Living Wellness

TABLE OF CONTENTS

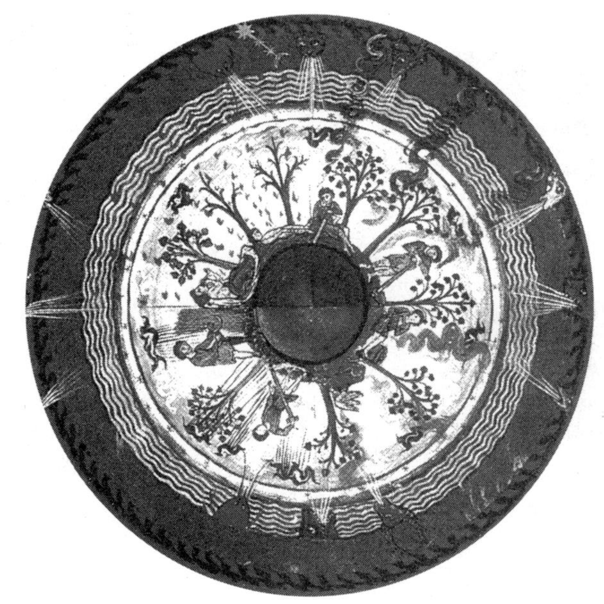

*"A wheel was shone to me, wonderful to behold...
Divinity is in its omniscience and omnipotence like a wheel, a
circle, a whole, that can neither be understood, nor divided, nor
begun nor ended."*
—HILDEGARD VON BINGEN

June, 1998

"Living Wellness", an annual directory and journal, informs you of the latest approaches in holistic health care and guides you to qualified practitioners. You'll find holistic medical doctors, acupuncturists, chiropractors, nutritionists and psychologists, as well as services to complement these medically oriented practices. The comprehensive health related resources in, "Living Wellness" allow you to make informed health decisions and meaningful lifestyle choices.

This directory and journal was born out of our desire to find holistic practitioners to help us with our own health needs and those of our family and friends. We initially experienced our access to the holistic community confined to word of mouth. The time availability of a few well known practitioners was limited by their already busy schedules. Wanting more choices inspired us to develop, "Living Wellness", a creative resource of holistic health professionals. In our search for these professionals, we found not only a nucleus of health providers, but an interconnected community dedicated to holistic approaches. This community is committed to caring for whole individuals while supporting their unique journeys towards complete health. Rather than diagnose illness or imbalance based on a particular symptom, this community seeks an expanded causal approach, encompassing individuals' total body-mind systems. Through complementary medicine, which brings together traditional Western methods of medical doctors and hospitals with alternative and Eastern methods, this community innovates to best serve us.

To best serve ourselves, we are also realizing the importance of taking responsibility for our own health. We're playing an active role in educating ourselves to make responsible choices about our physical, emotional, mental and spiritual well-being. We are no longer relying on quick, magic cure-alls from doctors, but instead hearing Nature's wisdom to know and care for our whole system's needs. We are becoming disease preventative to ensure our vitality. With access to the holistic health community, "Living Wellness" seeks to support us in making informed decisions about our health.

"Living Wellness" is meant to help each of us bring together a circle of practitioners who offer a sound basis for our healing and self awareness. These doctors, teachers, practitioners and artists together can help us realize and establish our expanded vision of health.

Sincerely yours,

The Editors

Soul Retrieval For Modern Medicine

Gayle Madeleine Randall, MD

Ancient philosophers, such as Plato and Aristotle and current authors have considered the existence of soul, but few have contemplated including soulfulness in the practice of modern medicine. Everybody would agree we live in a physical world and that diseases have physical relationships. However, we in the West rarely consider that diseases have relationship to soul. Viewing health through a sense of soulfulness gives us a greater understanding of how to alleviate disease.

Medicine, religion and magic all come from common roots in our ancient heritage. However, the dominance of 'techno-medicine' makes it fashionable to believe that medicine has nothing to do with our ancient heritage. Accordingly, most physicians do not fathom the true meaning of health and wholism. They tend to think of illness as based only in the physical body and have lost sight of wholism which is inclusive of physical, emotional, mental and spiritual bodies.

 How did we lose our souls to medical technology? As medical science advanced, and 'techno-diagnosis' became more available, doctors began to rely more heavily on science for the answers. Advanced training and physician specialization led doctors to look at patients as their diseases. 'Techno-medicine' increased the cost of health care in the U.S. astronomically. HMO's became popular, which stressed reducing costs by seeing more patients in less time. This development only further distanced physicians from the people they served and we lost that sacred connection.

Technology and science are potent healing tools, but we began to think technology was the spirit; and when we stopped honoring the spirit and began honoring only matter and technology, we lost something in our ability to heal. We lost access to the healing energies available to us through the unseen world. Unfortunately, most doctors either ignore or take energy for granted. But we can use energies, like those of the earth, for example, to heal ourselves and others.

How can one meld modern medicine with the realm of spirit? Shamans have maintained the essence of the healing priests of ancient times. The shaman understands that disease is the loss of equilibrium in the patient who is not living in harmony with the universal laws. The shaman heals by giving patients new hope which changes their perspective about the future and returns their power. This requires that the patient

Continued on page 5

Continued from page 4

take responsibility for their illness and understand that illness is a teacher. The shaman acts by helping to translate the message of the illness. Right within the illness is the gift of our own wholeness or health that can lead us back to balance.

In order to put the soul back into modern medicine, we need a current, scientifically relevant and soul-centered spiritual view. I have found that evaluating and treating the body, mind, emotionality and spirit, and using science and technology are all part of the same process.

This new paradigm for health is an integrative process of evaluation and treatment that moves far beyond the physical realm. In addition to Western Medicine, it is inclusive of guided meditation, prayer, color healing, dreaming, the Medicine Wheel and collaboration of practitioners from all healing traditions. This new structuring is returning the sacred nature to the healing professions and reclaiming medicine as a spiritual art as well as a science. ✱

A Better Birth

Alone, uninformed, unsupported and absolutely terrified... that's my memory of the births of my children. With contractions every three minutes, I drove myself to the hospital to give birth to my son. The doctor who "delivered" my daughter induced all of "his" births and told me I could choose for her to be born on a Friday or a Tuesday. That was the extent of my choices. I was shaved, given an enema, my bag of waters was ruptured and my labor was induced with pitocin. Then I was left alone. My husband wasn't allowed in the room during examinations or the birth. The nurse didn't believe me when I told her the baby was coming. The doctor arrived with barely enough time to take off his jacket and slip the gloves on his hands before my daughter made her entrance. What should have been the most beautiful moments in my life were lonely, frightening, and painful.

Wasn't birth supposed to be a joyful, loving, spiritual process, with some caring person by my side from early labor throughout the birth process... someone to provide support, answer my questions and reduce my anxiety... someone to encourage me to have the birth I'd always wanted, with comfort and caring and knowledge of birth to ease my fears?

The answer is YES — that 'someone' is a doula. With the support of a doula, birth can be more like it was for our grandmothers and great-grandmothers, but with the safety net of modern technology nearby. Doulas are women who provide continuous emotional and physical support for the mother and her partner at home, in a birth center or at the hospital. Doulas stay throughout the labor, regardless of the length, providing massage, a loving touch, heat and cold packs, a birth ball, and suggestions that encourage labor or help turn the baby into the proper position for delivery. Their presence has been shown to give the mother an easier, shorter labor, with less pain, a reduced chance of an unnecessary cesarean delivery, reduced use of anesthesia and analgesia, reduced need for drugs to stimulate labor's progress, and a safer, healthier birth and baby. And as an added benefit, the parent-infant attachment is enhanced even long after the birth.

I became a doula to help women experience the joy and beauty of giving birth, to give them the birth that I never had. To help the woman feel safe, loved, nurtured, and supported, so she can focus on managing her pain and bringing her baby safely into the world, and her partner can focus on loving her during the process. ✳

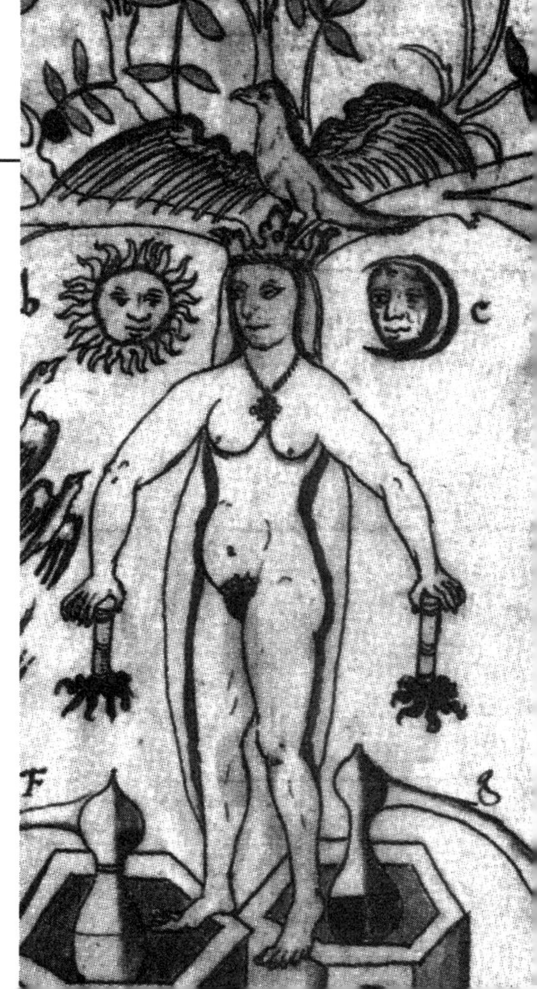

CALLING THE COUNCIL

Several years ago I was asked to speak about council to a group of seventy-five teachers and storytellers who were participating in a conference on the power of story. Midmorning of the first day, I found myself standing behind a traditional lectern, looking out over very straight rows of expectant faces. The incongruity of the situation stopped me cold. Rather than talking at them about council, I wanted to provide an experience of participating in one directly. But I had less than two hours and there weren't enough experienced council leaders at the conference to create smaller, more manageable groups. Introducing council for the first time to more than twenty people is a challenge. A council of seventy-five felt overwhelming!

In my moment of indecision, I remembered that a council leader's overriding commitment is to respond creatively to the moment. The situation may demand relinquishing familiar patterns in order to work with current realities in a productive way. So, throwing caution to the wind, I asked my audience to rearrange themselves in a large circle. The sound of scraping chairs dominated the next few minutes as I tried to come up with a plan that would allow seventy-five people the option to speak in the time allotted. Some might choose to be silent, but I needed a focus that would allow those who wanted to speak to do so — briefly, but in a satisfying way.

Sitting in the large circle brought me home. Immediately a workable plan and a suitable theme popped into my head. Unwrapping the carob pod talking stick I usually brought to such gatherings, I began:

"We're going to pass this large carob pod around the circle in a clockwise direction from person to person. Only the person holding the pod is allowed to talk. The rest of us listen as attentively as we can. The four intentions are; first, 'Speaking from the heart', second, 'Listening from the heart', third, 'Being of lean expression' and fourth, 'Spontaneity', meaning we speak without planning, 'what to say'. You may choose not to speak. Silence can make an important contribution to the circle. For this council I'd like you to tell a very short story about a shameful or embarrassing moment in your childhood — a story you haven't shared with many people, perhaps not even your immediate family or closest friends. Our circle is large, so choose your words carefully and relate just the essence of the story."

I decided to begin.

"Although my grandmother intimidated many people in our family, I was her favorite, which is probably one of the reasons I loved her so much. In my earliest memories, she already had a full head of white hair and the caustic sense of humor she took to the grave. Towards the end of her life we played hilarious games of gin rummy in the living room of her Atlantic City boarding house. When Nellie died, I experienced penetrating grief for the first time in my life."

"One of my greatest joys in those teenage years was playing a favorite piece of classical music on the phonograph while I 'conducted' the orchestra. After my mother told me the news of my grandmother's death, I closed the door of my bedroom and put on the slow movement of Beethoven's Seventh Symphony, a piece I knew would embrace my sadness. I was passionately drawing out the best from the New York Philharmonic, when my mother burst into the room. 'Shut it off!' she shouted over the music. 'In the Jewish tradition, you're not supposed to do anything joyous when a family member dies!' I thought playing a melancholy piece I loved dearly honored my grandmother, so the intensity of the rebuke left me confused and ashamed. I didn't know about the tradition and, besides, we could hardly be called observant Jews. I smoldered with injustice for days. My mother and I didn't have a chance to clear the air between us until a week after the funeral."

My story took less than a minute. Others followed in turn with their anecdotes, some funny, some sad, some mundane, some bizarre. A mood of relaxed attentiveness prevailed, which soon created a feeling of intimacy in the circle. One man took a few minutes to share something he had never told anyone. His tears were contagious. As it turned out, only one person passed the talking piece without speaking. When I finally took the large carob pod from the person on my right, I glanced at my watch. We had gone around the circle in one hour and twenty minutes. There was still time to have a discussion with a group of people who now felt at ease with each other and touched by the magic of council. ✴

Jack Zimmerman, "The Way of Council" (in collaboration with Virginia Coyle)

As I stood in front of a roomful of eager women, being retrained to re-enter the workforce after several years of motherhood, sharing my personal journey with cancer for the past five-plus years, I was completely immobilized by a sudden blanket of unbearable heat sweeping over my body. It was as though someone had instantly turned the temperature in the room up to about 100+ degrees! I felt my face flush with this high heat, droplets of perspiration covering my forehead, my entire body drenched with sweat. Two things immediately passed through my mind at the same moment: a sense of absolute embarrassment as I lost my train of thought; and an overwhelming fear that the cancer was again taking hold!

Marilyn Joyce, author of, "5 Minutes to Health".

MY JOURNEY TO MENOPAUSE NATURALLY

Though feeling sick in the pit of my stomach, somehow I made it through the rest of that day. Rushing home, I soon found solace in a warm tub. That night, I fell into a deep sleep, only to awaken in the middle of the night immersed in a cold swamp of sweat. I was utterly convinced that the cancer was back. I did not sleep a wink the rest of the night. The next morning, the pessimist that I had become, apprehensively picked up the phone and called the doctor, my voice trembling, tears running down my face, as I asked for an appointment as soon as possible.

As I related the circumstances of the previous day to my doctor, a young and rather impudent man, I could see that he was fighting hard not to burst into laughter. I angrily demanded to know why he seemed to experience such humor at my expense! He reached over, taking my hands in his, now openly laughing, as he jokingly asked me how I felt about, 'the change of life'. My confusion was apparent as I fumbled over questions about how this could be when I was not yet 40 years old. One part of me was tremendously relieved to know that it was not cancer revisited, while another part of me fell into a weeping mass at the thought of losing my womanhood so early and having to deal with the embarrassment of the day before on a regular basis.

As young and arrogant as I had perceived him to be, my understanding doctor compassionately explained that this was not the end of my womanhood, simply another phase. With a grocery list of books to look for, and supplements to consider, and an armful of pamphlets and booklets to read, I left the doctor's office. You see, as a uterine cancer survivor, I was not a candidate for hormone replacement therapy. In fact, even if I were, I would not have considered such. I wanted to deal with this as naturally as possible. So the research began.

I had already developed a very wholesome dietary and lifestyle regime in my journey back to wellness from cancer. However, I found myself asking, "What more can I do since I can't use HRT?" "What are the health risks associated with menopause?" & "Is there anything natural I can do to protect myself?"

First of all, the health risks included osteoporosis, heart disease, colon cancer, and vaginal dryness, the latter significantly diminishing sexual pleasure, Generally, with some planning around my food intake and lifestyle practices, it appeared that those fluctuating hormones could be very well controlled. Obviously,

however, something was missing in my regime. I quickly chose to view menopause, as I had a previous bout with cancer, my teacher.

I began to be aware of the things that triggered a hot flash or night sweat. These included hot drinks, hot meals (whether fire-hot or spice-hot), alcohol, a warm room, hot weather, a warm bed or an emotional upset. It became clear that the degree of depression, anxiety, dizzy spells or headaches varies from woman to woman, and in my life, from day to day! However, the misnomer was to believe that there was nothing I could do but suffer, or begin HRT. And, in my search for information regarding menopause, there were some key natural steps that I have regularly adopted into my lifestyle, which have successfully counteracted the negative impacts of menopause.

1) Get "back to basics" in your eating habits. Whole foods prepared simply, at least 50% of your vegetables and fruits eaten raw. Aim for 7-10 servings of vegetables per day and about 2-3 servings of fruit per day.

2) Include foods rich in phytoestrogens. They offer many of the benefits of HRT without the side effects. These plant chemicals are found in tofu, tempeh, soymilk, soybeans, alfalfa, flaxseeds, sunflower seeds, sesame seeds, yams, olive oil, parsley, garlic, papaya, chickpeas, and red beans.

3) Exercise daily. At least 1/2 hour per day of a natural form of exercise, preferably walking, swimming, cycling, swimming or dancing. Strap some light weights onto your wrists and ankles to got those extremities really working!

4) Allow time every day for relaxation. Take a yoga or Tai Chi class to assist you in gaining and maintaining a sense of inner calmness, centeredness and balance.

5) Join a women's support group. Having the support and sharing of others gives you the strength to get through the tough times.

So, to answer the question many of you are probably asking, No, I do not suffer with night sweats or hot flashes these days. And depression — well, I felt much more depression and anxiety during my youth than ever I do now. My life at this time is bountiful, joyful, extremely meaningful, and generally peaceful! ✳

Natural Allies *In Search of a Mentor*

By Stephen Johnson, Ph.D.

The mentor provides a bridge away from the father, guiding the young man to cut the parental ties.

"Mentor" first appears in Homer's Odyssey as a loyal adviser of Odysseus who was entrusted with the care and education of Odysseus' son, Telemachus. Throughout history, a mentor has been a wise and trusted counselor, usually at least 10 to 15 years older than his mentor or student. The mentor has skill and has performed his craft to a level of mastery. He, as an example or model, passes on his skill and shows the student how his dreams can be realized.

The mentor recognizes the meaningful issues in the student. He enhances the experience for the younger man who has already achieved something and is looking for more. The "Puer," which is Latin for "boy," is an uninitiated or naive male who longs for someone to acknowledge his gifts, to validate him and to bestow a blessing. The father often misses this opportunity, since the role of provider usually takes him away from the house. When the father is away, the house is turned over to the mentor.

It is not traditionally the father's job to see into his son's soul nor is it the mentor's job to put a roof over the boy's head or to protect him. The mentor provides a bridge away from the father, guiding the young man to cut the parental ties and bond with nature. The mentor sees the boy's spirit and gives him a name. He opens the world — of the boy's interest to and guides him in finding his direction.

My ally and best friend, genuine mentor for the first 19 years of my life, was my grandfather. His name was Lawrence Stewart, but everyone called him Stew. He was just that sort of a fellow, too, who would answer to a nickname like that. Scottish, 6'2", perpetually grinning, bald and rugged; he was bigger than life itself. He had a huge lap that could hold both me and his dog at the same time.

Stew was a man's man who loved the great outdoors and cherished fishing and hunting as expressions of his personal relationship with the wilderness and survival. He frequently wore moccasins, a deer hide jacket, suspenders and a broad brimmed hat.

He was a self-taught carpenter and an artist who had a shop in the back yard which served as a sacred container for his special creations. The shop had all the right tools and every size nail and screw and it was home for a vast array of paints and pastels of every hue. This space had no doubt been sanctified for a wizard to fashion the very things that would delight a young, aspiring apprentice.

As an ally, Stew accepted and validated me without question. He unconditionally loved me and I knew that I was pleasing to him. He admired me and always seemed curious and interested in what I was thinking, dreaming and doing. I could fantasize with him and we would tell tales, spin yarns, make up stories and even, on occasion, act them out.

As a mentor, he taught me to ride a horse, steer a boat, guide a plane, tie a fishhook and whittle a piece of wood. He encouraged me to go for it; not to hold back but to stretch and reach for what I wanted. I felt his support and knew that he stood behind what I was doing. This provided the needed safety to attempt the new, the daring or even the seemingly impossible. Unquestionably, I felt that he was on my side.

My grandfather served me in many ways; not least among them was providing a model of what a real friend and ally could be to another. He stood for loyalty and devotion. He displayed strength and courage. He was commanding while avoiding being demanding. He had a gentle side and even a frail side which I saw from time to time. His compassion and understanding always revealed the depth of his caring. He told me his truth and made room for mine.

He displayed the traits of a man who had grown up during the depression and had learned to make it on his own and fight for what he knew was right. As a high ranking Mason he embraced the same daring pioneer spirit that helped to guide the founding fathers of this country. He represented freedom to me; the freedom to be myself, no matter what.

Stew made an impact on me, leaving an impression that will be felt for my entire life. The legacy that he passed on has given me the courage to embark on the journey and the strength to endure the tests along the way.

I think the pain of his death was too overwhelming for me when I was 19, so I avoided truly grieving the loss until only a few years ago. It was in the midst of my midlife crisis that I finally allowed myself to realize how deeply I have missed him and how much I would have liked to have had his soothing support during such a challenging time in my life.

When I talk with other men, they frequently tell me stories about a special relationship with a grandparent or another elder. An honoring is expressed as they speak of their mentors with respect and appreciation.

However, there are countless numbers of young men in this country who are starving from father-hunger and who have never experienced the mutual admiration inherent in a mentoring relationship. Due to the breakdown of the nuclear family over the last 25 years, we have drifted apart and we are now suffering the pain of that alienation and isolation. We have a vast generation of men going through midlife crises together, longing for the wisdom and understanding of a ritual elder. These men are eager for the spiritual initiation into conscious manhood and are searching for greater understanding of what it means to be a balanced male in a changing world.

Additionally, with so much importance these days directed toward the young and the youthful lifestyle in this country, there's a growing tendency to ignore or even neglect our ritual elders as unpleasant reminders of aging and mortality. Many of our seniors have been passed over and have tended to lose sight of their own intrinsic worth.

I sincerely hope that we don't forget the inherent value of the grandfather in this regard as a natural resource; but, rather, commission our elders to pass on their history to our offspring. ✳

THIS BEATING HEART

by Caitriona Reed

The air is cold and damp. Clouds lie low on the mountains, hiding them from sight. Through the clouds I see patches of snow on the ridges. My feet are cold. It is mid-day. I live here. I have lived here for the past five years. I came here as a man. Now I am a woman.

I came to establish a retreat center, far enough away from the cities of Southern California to give to the people who come here a sense of space, of the land, of being in a particular place with a particular history, particular plant and animal inhabitants, a climate consisting of four distinct seasons.

I came here to grow — as a teacher, and as a person. This cold wind from the north, the aftermath of another big winter storm, chills me. It excites me too. Even though my body is cold, I feel relaxed and safe. It's hard to imagine the stillness of summer; the heat, the intoxicating air, heavy with chamise and sage.

I don't know what it is to be a man. I don't know what it is to be a woman. They are two words we use with such ease, and such a vast array of assumptions. People say that within the cultural framework of our ancient, collective, palleolithic past, there were people like myself — not man, not woman. Some say we were healers and shamans. The anthropologists and missionaries used us as examples to prove their various points. It's enough for me to know that there have always been others willing to ask questions in order to be true to themselves.

I've been called a teacher — of Buddhism, Meditation, the Dharma — for seventeen years now. People I have great regard for have, to my amazement, acknowledged me as such. Now, tired of words, excited about my new life, I choose to question even that.

Amidst all the changes, it is this call to question everything that surprises me the most. I have fewer answers than ever, and it is as refreshing as the February wind, fierce and dangerous, blowing away what is stale and contrived. I am unwilling to compromise, or to waste a single moment of my life. Suddenly, I trust the landscape inside me as much as I trust the mountains and the wind — kindness, fear, fearlessness, impatience, joy...all of it.

I thought, as a transsexual teacher, I would be throwing away my credibility and my dignity, to become a mere curiosity. Instead, I discovered resources of strength I never knew existed. It's not that I wanted to challenge things for the sake of challenging them. I have no patience for mere contentiousness.

In this time of trees burning by the tens of thousands of square kilometers, of the gunfire we pretend not to hear, of the despair we maintain is not our own, of the children eaten alive by the violence that surrounds us...none of us can afford to hide the truth for a moment, no matter what is costs, and none of us can afford not to ask questions.

Despite this, because of this, all my instincts are telling me that our liberation really is available, right here and now, in our honoring of this beating heart, these eyes seeing, this body dancing, not resting in contrived truths, not afraid to ask the questions — here and now, or nowhere else at all. ✴

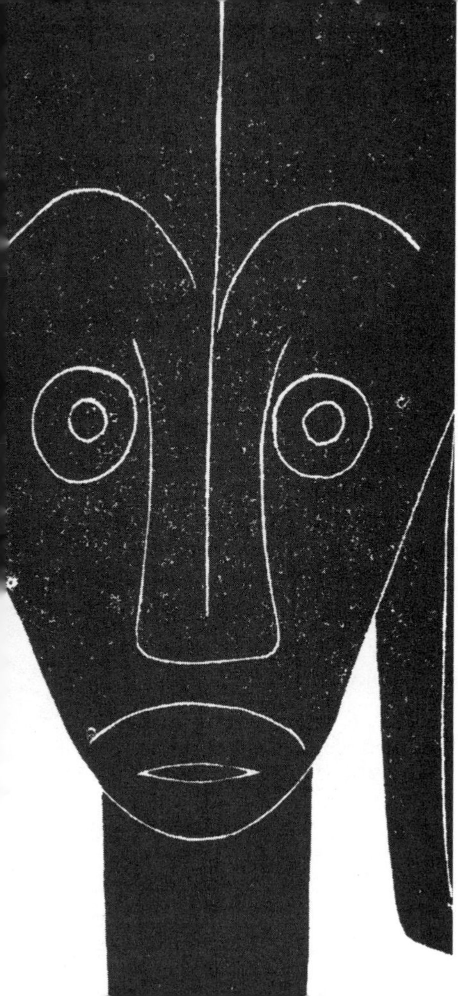

ILLNESS AS TRANSFORMATION

by Maryana Palmer, M.A., M.F.C.C.

I've been working with cancer patients for twenty years now, and I still continue to be awed and inspired by people's strength and courageous spirit. It is truly a blessing to be part of their journey, a journey that is indeed very powerful.

When you are initially diagnosed with cancer, your life becomes a whirlwind. It is very common to feel hopeless, despairing, confused and very vulnerable. Suddenly and abruptly, you are faced with a crisis that affects your total being and often for the first time you are facing your mortality. Over night you are truly thrown into facing a "dark night of the soul."

Continued on page 15

It is often at this very time of crisis that people hunger for new meanings, new ways to understand suffering. It is my belief that dark nights of the soul can become initiations into a new way of being. This time of intense transition can offer the opportunity to reflect on our lives deeply and respond to the crisis that faces us. When a patient is willing to embark on this journey and respond to the darkness then a life-affirming newness can emerge.

The healing process of this journey is difficult to explain, because it is so very different and unique for each individual based on their histories and yet there are some common parameters. Most people I work with embrace a holistic approach to health combining traditional medicine and alternative methods. The illness sparks a strong desire to mobilize their self-healing abilities and do all they can to strengthen their immune systems. Recognizing the important connection of mind, body and spirit, they begin to explore their lives on these three levels, the physical, psychological, and the spiritual. The physical level consists of nutrition, medicine, exercise and movement programs. The psychological and spiritual levels bring us back to the dark night of the soul. When people are willing to face the pain then a deep psycho-spiritual exploration can begin. In individual therapy and/or support groups, they are able to explore areas of stress and old beliefs and patterns that may have kept them unhappy or stuck in their lives or perhaps just neutral. Through this process, leading to increased awareness and empowerment, they are able to transform patterns and move beyond past conditioning, the dullness of repression and the old familiar ways of life to find themselves in new territory. They begin to understand reality more clearly and deeply. A new self develops, more passionate and alive than the self they once were.

A necessary and meaningful part of this process includes people learning to take control of their own lives and truly searching for lifestyles that are meaningful and joyful to them. No longer are their lives oriented by others "shoulds" but rather by what's important to them. The journey often intensifies the search for what is most sacred in life and people begin to expand and clarify their own unique spiritual paths. They begin to see the broader picture of life, perspectives change and new priorities emerge. There is a focus on quality of life moment to moment, because cancer patients realize there are no guarantees for any of us and the moment is all we have.

When one embarks on this path, there is a gradual completion of unfinished business, a releasing of stress, and an openness to more joy and the fullness of life. No one wants a diagnosis of cancer, but if one is open and able to respond, it can offer the opportunity for deep transformation leading to a richer, more fulfilling life. A life blessed with wisdom and grace that is an inspiration to all of us. ✴

QUANTUM LEAP

CREATIVITY TO HEALTH

Philip D'Arbanville

To create stability of health and balance for ourselves, our families and our communities, we need to synthesize our scientific, philosophical, and religious wisdom, with the creative expression of our own internal truth. Unless we marry our perceptions of reality with our inner experience consciously, we will continue to perpetuate a conflicting duality of self. The outer personality will continue to operate on old patterns of understanding, while our true sense of self remains unable to come to terms with new feelings and thoughts. The stress of this conflict eventually results in disease affecting our emotional, mental, or physical well-being.

This conflict is a natural result of our evolving consciousness. Quick changes in this time push us beyond our limits. We fail to process through our dreaming state into our conscious awareness all that is thrust upon us. Instantaneous, worldwide media coverage pounds tons of new content into us daily. We're constantly, redefining reality through quantum, astro and meta-physics. This forces us to reach deeper into our own psyche to come to terms with who we are and what our new purpose is. Without processing all this new awareness, we develop illnesses. Like the undigested meal, our psyche-mind-body doesn't fully assimilate our experiences. This results in increased nervousness, stress and finally depression. We continue the spiral into further depression by taking symptom relieving drugs like Prozac. What other real solutions do we have? Creativity might hold the key.

The artistic process provides the expression of that which we yearn for...in fact, our whole selves. Modern man/woman, fully conscious of the present, affords us this unique vision. Artists explore deeper levels of Self and through struggle and sacrifice, give birth to that which has yet to find expression. We all benefit to some degree by

Continued on page 17

Continued from page 16

witnessing and exploring the artist's shared vision, which in turn stimulates our own creative process.

The artist is not unlike the cutting edge scientist delving into her/his quantum experiment or the philosopher struggling with ancient Vedic text. It's a mutual quest to know that which is yet to "exist" in our conscious mind. The creative urge works to reveal what we sense inside us as a disquieting rumble shaking our foot-hold on 'Self'.

To Quest is to embark on the mythic journey paradigm as presented by Joseph Campbell; wherein one breaks from society, takes an inward retreat deep into the realms of the psyche, has a confrontation with challenging images & forces, conquers and assimilates new realities into the conscious mind and returns to society with an increased power of perspicuity and the ability to share insights with humanity.

We who yearn to experience life to the fullest, all sooner or later embark consciously on our journey to come into our own, to actualize more of our higher potential. Expression through any chosen medium such as paint, sculpture, words, dance, music, story, theater or film, is the attempt to expose that which we've recovered from the inner sanctum of our nature and thereby complete our journey through sharing the vision and being witnessed in the process. Since our inner growth evolves endless cycles of becoming, we are impelled, after a period of rest, to journey yet again into more of the 'unknown' and wrestle with our demons and gods to extract further portions of Self from our own great mystery.

Art venues exhibit other's creative processing and expression. How deeply we absorb images, in all their content and purpose, determines to what degree we ourselves are inspired. When we awaken energies by association, our own creative process gets nudged towards action. Of course, no one can jump start the process for us. Each individual makes his/her own choice to Self-explore and eventually share their insights through some art form. As required school art programs show, no matter how much fun we may have, we're not ready to embark on our own odyssey until the need strikes us. It has to well up from within, strongly enough for us to make it a priority.

The artistic process itself is an essential developmental formula for self birth into our full humanness. All of us, regardless what our level of so called "natural ability or talent", need to employ our own creative process if we are to reach towards the full expression of our nature; in short, to realize a deep sense of value from living our life. No less important than physical exercise, healthy cuisine, or spiritual discipline, is our knowledge of how to engage our creative process. Our creative acts fulfill our soul's yearning for expression and prime the causal level of our being, our "raison d'être" in the first place.

"Health", the homeostasis of our complex system from physical to meta physical, is as much a result of inner processing as outer lifestyle choices. We all know of purist vegans who've succumbed to life threatening diseases. Yes, earth, air, water, sound, and mind pollution all bombard our systems and we can lay the blame at the feet of industrialized waste led by corporate greed. Yet our health is always about our choices, on all levels. Victimization is merely self-imposed apoplexy. We can choose to remain ignorant or to educate ourselves, to drink polluted water or natural spring water, to live in high risk radiation zones or rural environments, all depending on the priorities we've established or merely passively accepted for ourselves. Lest we forget, even choosing not to choose is a choice. We can become active choice makers, take responsibility for our fate and work to help create clean, healthy environments, healthy food and better schools. Life itself, when completely valued, impels us to take such actions as the practical application of insights gleaned from our individual creative processes.

Artistic process then, from this perspective, is the quantum leap we as individuals can take to process our whole nature into self-conscious awareness.

Artistic process then, from this perspective, is the quantum leap we as individuals can take to process our whole nature into self-conscious awareness. This facilitates balance in our inner and outer worlds, — our emotional, mental, and physical states. With this new balance, we can evolve more of our potential and become more involved in our outer worlds for the better. This brings ourselves, our families and ultimately our communities more balance and complete health. From this point of view, health is a state of condition, always in motion, flux, change... a vital balance of interdependent systems... never an end reached unto itself, but a shared state of equilibrium propelled into ever increasing challenges as we grow in potential expression. It is life itself. ✳

THE PRACTITIONERS AND PROVIDERS

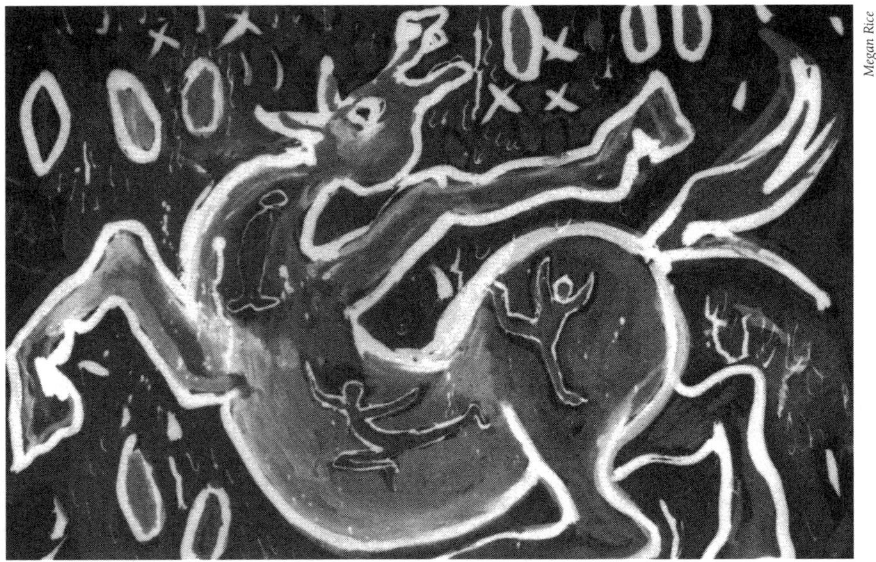

"Imagination is more important than knowledge"
—ALBERT EINSTEIN

ARTS/CREATIVITY EXPERIENTIAL WORKSHOPS & PERFORMANCE, DANCE, MUSIC, PAINTING, SCULPTURE & THEATRE

In our endeavor to make meaning of life and the world around us, art encourages expression of self beyond customary patterns, and advances our creativity. Art opens and engages our sensorial, tactile and imaginal worlds, offering access to our whole mind-body instrument and its innate knowing of health. Art creates an opportunity for fuller communication of thought, intuition, feeling and spirituality.

Aparecida

Sacred Sensual Body. Transformation, empowerment and healing through Belly Dance and Ritual. Classes on Thursday nights at West Side Academy of Dance 7:45-9:30 pm. Workshops, private sessions and performances. See ad page 69
1711 Stewart Ave.
Santa Monica, CA   (310) 712-3925

Sarah Berges

Contemporary Dance for adults and Creative Dance for children to stimulate body, mind, & heart toward self awareness & creative interplay with the world.
See ad page 76
Santa Monica   (310) 396-7324

Radha Carman
Teacher & Performer

Kerala Dance Theatre offers classes and performances in Mohini Attam & Kathakali, the Dance Theatre of India.
See ad page 90
          (310) 837-8568

Myrna Castaline

A Mask Making Journey: Masks serve as a bridge from ordinary consciousness to non-ordinary, powerful states which are alive within our psyches. As we make a mask of our own face, we tap into a flow of creative wisdom that awakens within us the inherent powers of self-healing and transformation. Letting the mask speak to us and through us deepens our understanding of self. See ad page 76
          (310) 455-3223

Mathew Cohen

Sacred Power Movement: Move from the secular to the sacred to the sacred natural grace. Develop more energy, power, and vitality with Chi Gong, Chi Gong breath, sound, dance and Yoga. Twenty years in Martial Arts, Dance and other body-mind disciplines, Mathew has a Martial Arts and Massage practice in Santa Monica and teaches internationally. See ad page 77
Santa Monica

          (310) 392-6788

Continuum sm

Continuum inquires into our capacity to participate in the health and well-being of ourselves. See ad page 91
http://home.earthlink.net/~continuummove
1629 18th St. #7, Santa Monica, CA   90404
          (310) 453-4402

Lynn Creighton

The sculptural forms that come through her enact the feminine, becoming fully aware of itself and its ability to re-create and to celebrate life. See ad page 74
Northridge   (818) 886-9006

Adornments of Desire
Carla Cummings

Henna rituals for rites of passage, festivals and energy shifts. Custom jewelry for energy alignments.
Los Angeles   (323) 651-6461

Dancing Women, Mary Donovan

Goddess, spirit, dancing soul. Empowerment. Playshops. A world of celebration of female wholeness and holiness. Friday classes.
1629 18th St. Santa Monica, CA   90404
          (310) 828-8073

Explore into Character
Theatre for the Soul
Philip & Michele D'Arbanville

Using authentic gesture, ancient text, and spoken word, together we will create a bridge for the imaginal worlds to be felt and witnessed. A gateway of expression for our personal and mythic stories,

Continued

this workshop offers improvisation and exploratory process for anyone who yearns to deepen their creative expression.
See ad page 85
Topanga & Westside   *(310) 455-2714*

The FLM Art Studio
Francette Louise Mace: Intense, explorative work towards full expression of creativity, using color, movement, dreamwork, and storytelling in the medium of painting and sculpture. All levels welcome.
francettelouise@hotmail.com
Los Angeles   *(310) 837-7147*

Ruth Gould Goodman
L.Ac., M.A. Dance Therapy
Movement Essentials Studio: Bone by Bone, Breath by Breath, Head to Toe activate your intention to be Vitally Healthy and Beautiful. Learn to EmBody the Joy, Power and Creativity of the present moment through this unique yoga of mindful movement and voicing.
See ad page 75
Venice & Mar Vista
        (310) 392-3612 or (310) 395-5504

Mad Spirit
New Renaissance Folk Music Ensemble: Entertainment for celebrations, festivities, occasions. Music lessons also available.
Greater L.A. Area   *(310) 313-3084*

Kara Masters, M.A.
Registered Dance Therapist
In Touch: a practice of moving from the core to experience the resources of health, communication, creativity and joy inherent in your own dance. See ad page 82
Westside   *(310) 359-5599*

Meta Hara Presents
Personalized feminine spiritual movement facilitated by Thomai. Group or individual sessions available.
Topanga, Malibu & Pacific Palisades
        (310) 724-3246

Megan Rice
Art and Creativity classes for adults and children, given at "The Art Studio."
See ad page 89
115 S. Topanga Canyon Blvd.
Topanga, CA   90290   *(310) 455-2901*

Aryeh Shell, Dancing in the Tao
Communal celebrations and private healing explorations through sensation, movement, emotion, and psyche.
See ad page 125
Santa Monica   *(310) 939-3408*

Soundworks
Kabbalah Bernadette Bach
Sessions — private/ group. Tibetan instruments available. Inner quiet, personal wisdom with the sound of the Gongs.
See ad page 85
Los Angeles   *(310) 455-0063*

Robin Bush Vance, A.T.R., M.F.C.C.
Image-making is a visceral, into-the-blood stream language which provides a unique vocabulary for self understanding and creative insight. As an art therapist, I guide you in this process. See ad page 93
West Los Angeles & Pasadena
        (310) 281-7641

The Will Geer
Theatricum Botanicum
Situated in the Santa Monica Mountains, Theatricum offers classical summer repertory theatre, classes for Adults, Teens, and Youth, and award-winning educational outreach programs including School Days Field Trip Program and Classroom Enrichment. See ad page 78
1419 N. Topanga Canyon Blvd.
Topanga, CA   90290
(310) 455-2322 Box Office (310) 455-3723

BREATHWORK

Breathing is an involuntary physical function we can choose to slow, to quicken, to change. Conscious breathing unifies body and mind in the present moment. Becoming aware of our breath, one of the fundamental keys to life, can help release emotional blocks, toxins in the physical body and stress, as well as lower heart rate and reduce blood pressure.

Gail Darwin, CTF

The breath can be used to permanently detoxify the body, increase energy, clarity and focus, resolve old issues whether mental or emotional, and connect you with your soul in a very profound way. In my lifetime, as quickly as I can, I want to open the lungs of as many people as possible.

Santa Monica　　　　　　**(310) 656-0527**

Segan Elliott, M.A.

Living True Therapeutics, Conscious Breathwork/Spiritual Practitioner.
See ad page 98

Westside　　　　　　**(310) 397-9515**

"The real voyage of discovery consists not in seeking new landscapes, but in having new eyes"

—MARCEL PROUST

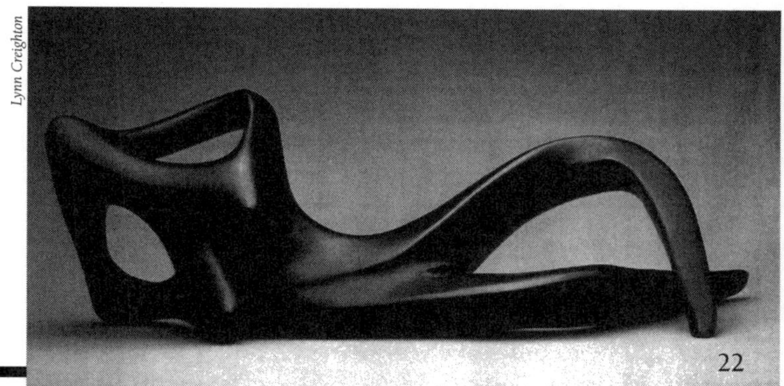

COLOR THERAPY
AURA-SOMA

Color Therapy and Aura-Soma are based on the belief that life force energy centers, called chakras, resonate to particular wavelengths of color. When people feel "off color," their chakras are out of balance. Color therapists and Aura-Soma practitioners offer non-intrusive, self-selective color systems which contain color, herbal and/or crystal energies for renewing harmony and well-being to the body, mind and spirit.

Ayn Cates

The Miracle of Color to take you on a journey to yourself. Private consultation, workshops, practitioner courses, astrology and products. See ad page 83

Santa Monica   (310) 578-5507

Lourdes Chazaro

I work with color puncture therapy, a gentle, non-invasive way of balancing your chakras, body, mind and spirit. See ad page 102

By appointment   (310) 358-6125

Catherine Engel

Bottles of luminous oils speaking to us in their language of color, Light, fragrance and Soul frequencies; Let's heal together. See ad page 69

Hollywood & Westside   (310) 459-4528

Healing Waters

Jennifer Otto

A place for healing, providing flower essences and AuraSoma color therapy; as well as a resource center for healing workshops and practitioners.

Los Angeles & Westside   (323) 651-4656

Institute for Health

Teresa Rispoli, L.Ac., Ph.D.
Color therapy has been scientifically proven. Certain colors affect our moods, temperament and feelings of well-being. See ad page 99

28247 Agoura Rd.
Agoura Hills, CA   91301

(818) 707-3126 (818) 707-2787 FAX

Fred Thompson, Aura-Soma USA

Conducting seminars in Los Angeles and world-wide, Fred Thompson's objective is to play within the powerful, creative energies connected within the sacred elements of color, sound, crystal and rhythm. He aims to facilitate the realization of sympathetic resonance with the essence of these archetypes through the process of internal and external alignment. See ad page 88

P.O. Box 88039, World Way Centre
Los Angeles, CA   90009

(310) 306-6265

COUNSELING PSYCHOTHERAPY PSYCHIATRY

*T*hese psychiatrists, psychotherapists and counselors bring a commitment to the integration of our spiritual, mental, emotional and physical states of consciousness. In addition, they bring their expertise in various disciplines, encompassing transformational and depth psychology; Jungian therapy; dream work; spiritual psychiatry; Buddhist practice; feminist therapy; Marriage, Family and Child practice; substance abuse recovery; HIV/AIDS counseling; energy healing; and meditation.

Valerie Benveniste, Ph.D.
Gentle transformational psychology for couples, individuals, children and adolescents. Psycho-educational and developmental assessments. See ad page 122
Westchester *(310) 240-1444*

Sylvia Bercovici, Ph.D.
Buddhist wisdom and meditation practice can help us realize our innate potential. See ad page 107
Santa Monica & West L.A. *(310) 470-1198*

Richard B. Cohen, M.F.C.C.
Innovative psychiatric and chemical dependency treatment. See ad page 98
Westside & Topanga *(310)455-4282*

G. Lynn Diamond, M.Ed., M.F.C.C.
Loss, spiritual issues, adolescents, couples and family work.
West Los Angeles *(310) 391-4088*

Patty Factor, M.F.C.C.
Therapeutic hikes enhance the experience of health, vitality, support and connection through nature and the group process. Children's, teen-age, and women's group hikes are offered, also individual, parent/child and family hikes. Call for more information and brochure. See ad page 110
Westside *(310) 588-0786*

Lillian Freeman, L.C.S.W.
Specializing in children ages 2 - 12, adolescents, family therapy, and individual counseling. Depression. Transitions. Career changes.
520 S. Sepulveda Blvd. L.A., CA 90049
  (310) 440-1963

Richard Gottfried, M.A., M.F.C.C.
Relationships, Parenting and Families, Loss and Change, Healing and Growth. Resolve relationship issues, address work concerns, handle parenting challenges, overcome depressed or anxious feelings due to loss or confusion. Mr. Gottfried draws upon his years of experience working with adults and families to provide a healing approach especially suited to the needs of each client. He is also a certified mediator.
21070 W. Summit Road
12381 Wilshire Blvd., Suite 200
Topanga *(310) 455-3804*
West Los Angeles *(310) 572-4366*

Judith Harte, Ph.D.

Depth Psychotherapist/Astrologer often incorporates Mythic Astrology within counseling sessions. See ad page 109

Westside & Sherman Oaks

(310) 281-7991

Alice Kagan, M.D.

Board Certified Psychiatrist

Wholistic and General Psychiatry and Energy Healing. See ad page 95

Beverly Hills & West Los Angeles

(818) 327-9952

Yona Kollin, L.C.S.W., B.C.D.

Concentrated healing as the foundation for emotional growth results in a healthy, fulfilling life. Psychotherapy, hypnotherapy, pain management, stress reduction, communication skills, relationship counseling, parenting issues, loss/grief counseling for all ages, individuals and couples. See ad page 91

Pasadena & Torrance *(626) 791-4547*

Men's Center of Los Angeles

Counseling and programs for individuals, couples, families and groups. Integrative approaches to psychotherapy... developing mind, body and spirit for men and the significant relationships in their lives.

Conscious living brings healthier functioning and greater fulfillment. See ad page 113

Woodland Hills/Beverly Hills

(818) 348-9302

Maryana Palmer, M.A., M.F.C.C.

Psychotherapy - mind, body, spirit - specializing in life-threatening illness, visualization, and bereavement. See ad page 72

520 S. Sepulveda Blvd. West L.A., CA 90049

(310) 455-1743

Margaret Paul, Ph.D.

InnerBonding Facilitator, Author, Speaker, Seminar Leader, Consultant. Individual, Couple, and Group Sessions - Business Consulting - Lectures/Workshops, 5-Day Intensives. *InnerBonding* is a powerful six-step mind/body/spirit healing process that will transform your life by teaching you how to: Establish a deep, daily personal connection and dialogue with Divine guidance. Free your essence, your core Self, the light within. Fill your heart with love and release creativity. Heal the false beliefs of your wounded self that cause fear, pain, addiction and relationship problems. Develop a powerful adult self who can take loving action and set loving boundaries for yourself and with others. See ad page 92
www.innerbonding.com

Los Angeles

(310) 390-5993 or (888) 6INNERBOND

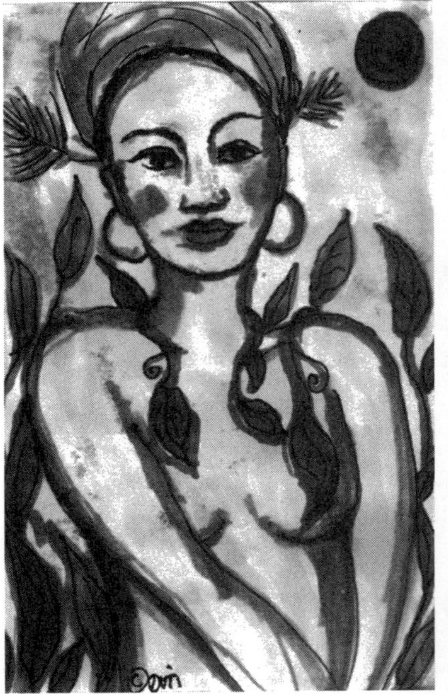

Outi Harma

"He alone is modern who is fully conscious of the present."

—Carl G. Jung

Michael George Philips, Ph.D.

Emotional healing through mirror reflection work. New Decision Therapy releases trauma and pain. A simple, easy approach with deep lasting benefits.

Los Angeles Valley　　　*(818) 360-4871*

Linnea Richards

Jungian therapy, dreamwork, hypnotherapy, family support, divorce therapy, parenting groups and educational tutoring.

Topanga & Los Angeles　　*(310) 455-2615*

Gina Ross, M.F.C.C.

Self-understanding and spiritual growth through a blend of Eastern and Western wisdoms and tools. Cross-cultural therapy in English, French, Spanish, Portuguese, Hebrew, Arabic and Italian. Trauma healing with EMDR, Somatic Experiencing, Emotional/Freedom Technique, and Reichian Bodywork. Couples work and Kabbalistic and Jungian principles. Serene garden setting.

L.A., Hancock Park　　　*(323) 930-2151*

Nancy L. Saks, Ph.D.

Holistic approach to adult, individual and couple psychotherapy to potentiate greater authenticity and connection with self and others. Bereavement counseling, stress management and issues related to significant life transitions and challenges.

Studio City & Beverly Hills

(818) 783-1900

Sharon Siegel, Ph.D., M.F.C.C.

Bereavement, death and dying work. Substance abuse recovery. HIV/AIDS counseling. Marriage, Family and Child counseling. Feminist and pre and post menopausal work. Mental health services. See ad page 116

Los Angeles　　　*(310) 455-3232*

Ginny Winn, M.F.C.C.

Heal relationships to - self - loved ones - work; mind & body, dream & shadow work; creative processes; brief solution-focused. Experience includes supervising interns at Antioch University Counseling Center & in elementary school. Fair fees.

P.O. Box 1275, Pacific Palisades, CA 90272

(310) 302-1139

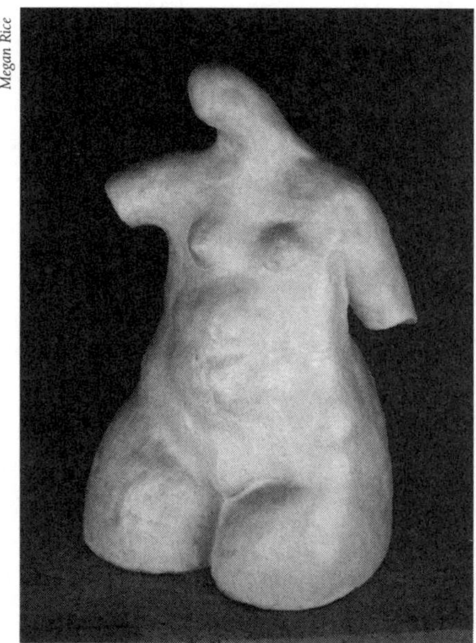

Megan Rice

"There is a vitality, a life force, an energy, a quickening, that is translated through you into action, and because there is only one of you in all time, this experience is unique. And if you block it, it will never exist through any other medium and will be lost."

—Martha Graham

ENVIRONMENTAL INTERIOR/ EXTERIOR DESIGN & CONSULTING

Environmental interior and exterior designers and consultants promote healthy, earth conscious and toxic-free choices for interior design, remodeling and new construction of homes and workplaces.

Green Clean

Environmentally correct house cleaning. Non-toxic products. Special ULPA allergy service. Meticulous, caring staff.
See ad page 84
greenguy@earthlink.net
Los Angeles   *(310) 385-7677*

Tim Ellis Constructions

General contractor committed to not using old growth trees. Specializing in seismic resistant construction and hillside construction. Recycles all usable waste. Utilizing newest technology in wood product engineering to reduce impact on the remaining native environment.
See ad page 96
tellis1@earthlink.net
                    (310) 455-0020

Ecology by Design

Audrey Hoodkiss

Interior design employing eco-safe materials & procedures to ensure a toxic-free & healthy indoor environment. Specialists in creating beautiful, harmonious & healing spaces. Supplier of environmental products.
626 Santa Monica Blvd. Suite 73
Santa Monica, CA   90401
                    (310) 394-4146

Forrest Painter Design

Constance Forrest, Psy.D.

Interior and landscape design. Psychological and human factors. See ad page 72
226 Sherman Canal
Venice, CA   90291
                    (310) 822-3640

John Gary Wallis, Architect

4 balanced sculptural architecture that is born out of the souls of the site and users. Call for consultation.
Global   *(310) 827-7854*

"Earth does not belong to us We belong to the earth"
—Chief Seattle

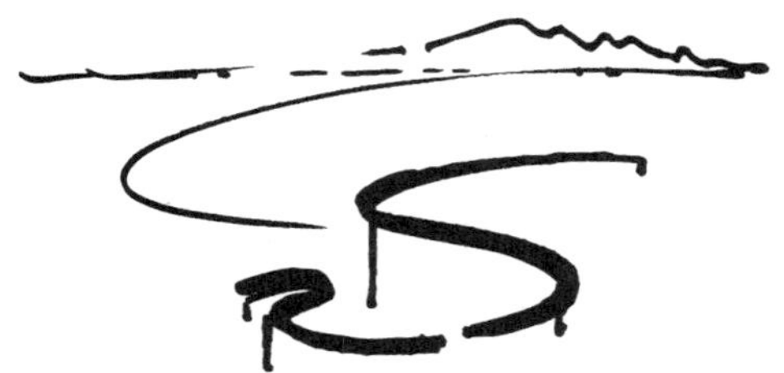

FENG SHUI

*P*racticed in China for thousands of years, Feng Shui is the environmental art of placement that harmonizes our energies with the earth's as well as the universe's rhthyms. Living and work spaces seek a balance of yin and yang while freely moving "chi" energy supports health, happiness and prosperity.

Kartar Diamond

Certified Feng Shui Consultant
*Feng Shui Solutions: Ancient Wisdom
for Better Modern Living*
Improve your home and work environment with ancient energetic principles of design and placement. Your physical surroundings impact your health, success, and relationships. Have a traditionally-trained specialist help you harness the opportunities and balance that you deserve. Long-distance internet clients welcome.
See ad page 77
http://www.loop.com/~kartar
Southern California   *(310) 820-7891*

Angi Ma Wong

Enjoy natural, holistic, empowered living by energizing your home and workplace through horoscope-customized consultations.
See ad page 122
Throughout the U.S.   *(310) 541-8818*

HEALTH INSURANCE

*A*s more people experience the value of holistic medicine, insurance companies are beginning to offer coverage for various practices, including acupuncture, chiropractic, craniosacral therapy, homeopathics, herbal remedies, psychological and spiritual counseling.

Continued

Michael Augello

Insurance Brokers for Health, Long Term Care and Life. We have plans that help pay for Alternative Medicine, Christian Science Nursing Providers, and Life Insurance for HIV+. We also have all the standard plans.
See ad page 104
Los Angeles, Southern California

(310) 455-0762

Jon Fazakerley, Insurance Agent & Estate Planning

Call for free consultation on policy evaluations, estate considerations, all types of coverage analysis. Health, Life, Alternative & Standard Plans.
See ad page 74
L.A., Southern California

(310) 854-0379

"To teach is to learn twice"
—JOSEPH JOUBERT

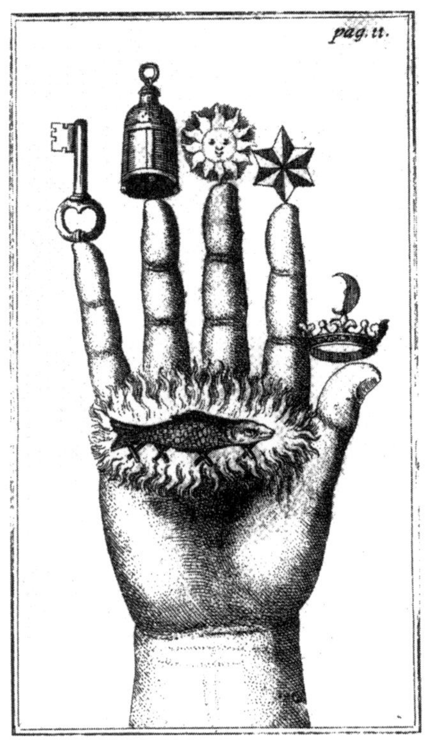

HOLISTIC ANIMAL CARE/WILD LIFE CENTERS

Animals, our closest companion souls in the evolutionary chain on earth, receive holistic care and health treatment, encompassing principles of non-shock, non-invasive, system-enhancing and balancing therapy. Acupuncture, herbal remedies, chiropractic and naturopathic procedures compliment traditional Western Veterinary medical care. Caregivers stress disease preventive, health preserving approaches.

Carol Alohalani Becker

Reiki Master & Animal Communicator

My communication and energy work facilitate spiritual, emotional and physical harmony in animals and people.
See ad page 117
Los Angeles area   **(323) 665-4222**

Holistic Veterinary Healthcare

Dr. Marc Bittan, D.V.M.

Acupuncture, Herbs, Homeopathy, Chiropractic. Special interest in Geriatrics, Acute & Chronic Disorders. See ad page 96
11673 National Blvd., L.A. CA 90064
     (310) 231-4415   (310) 231-4418 FAX

The Nature of Wildworks

Mollie Hogan

A rustic canyon care center, where wonderful animals of the wild are rescued, loved and cared for under an ongoing program in Topanga Canyon. Educational events and visits encouraged. Call for schedule. See ad page 105
Santa Monica Mountains   **(310) 455-0550**

Letisha Isabella

Holistic Health Care: Natural preventative dental care for pets using massage, music & herbs. No biters please. See ad page 95
Pasadena to Santa Barbara
     (800) 329-5495

Donald C. Kelliher, D.C.

Animal chiropractic practiced with an emphasis on chronic conditions. We revitalize normal biochemical function and revive uninterrupted nerve flow to the tissues. Full health restored.
Malibu, Agoura & Beverly Hills
     (310) 457-2047   (818) 707-6006

Dr. Sandy's Home Veterinary Care

Sandy Jongeward, D.V.M., Diplo. A.C.V.I.M.

No anesthesia dentals. Board Certified. Specialist of Internal Medicine.
Home calls   **(818) 708-7387**

Pat McKay Inc., Animal Nutrition

Pat McKay Inc. is devoted to giving you the information, products and services necessary for feeding your cats and dogs, the way Mother Nature intended. Fresh, wholesome, raw foods. See ad page 100
PatMcKay@GTE.nethttp://home1.GTE.net/PatMcKay
396 West Washington Blvd., Suite 600
Pasadena, CA 91103
     (626) 296-1120

Marty Meyer

Telepathic Animal Communication. Readings on pets by telephone. Behavior problems, conflicts, etc.
8728 Nye Rd. Ventura, CA 93001
     (805) 649-0720

Pets Naturally, Health Food & Supplies

One of the finest holistic resource centers for animal health products.
See ad page 104
Sherman Oaks   **(818) 784-1233**

Nancy Scanlan, D.V.M.

Monday and Tuesday 2:00p.m.-8:00p.m. and Wednesday 10:00a.m.-5:00p.m.
13624 Moorpark St.
Sherman Oaks, CA 91423
     (818) 784-9977

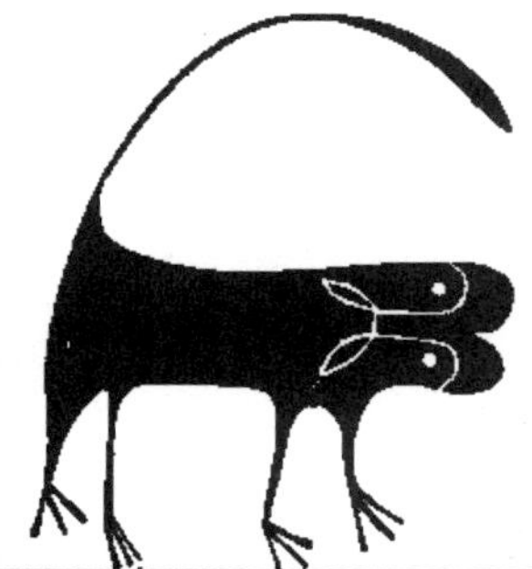

"The dog is the only being that loves you more than you love yourself"
—Fritz von Unruh

HOLISTIC PHARMACIES

Holistic pharmacies provide prescriptions from Homeopathic, Oriental Medical, Naturopathic and Ayurvedic Doctors as well as Herbalists. Prescriptions include tinctures and herbal mixtures in capsule or pill form; these non-allergenic, non-toxic healing remedies recharge your own immune system and expunge imbalancing elements from physical and electromagnetic levels. Holistic remedies are often less expensive than those from pharmaceutical companies as well as less toxic.

Acacia: Home Healthcare Center

Homeopathy, Herbs, Flower Essences.
4362 Fountain Ave. L.A., CA   90029

(800) 900-1600

Capitol Drugs

Capitol Drugs provides the communities we serve with a unique combination of full-service pharmacy, homeopathics, herbs, nutrition, aromatherapy, flower essences, sports nutrition, and more. Our trained staff is ready to guide you through this exciting variety of health care options. Too busy or too far away? We'll deliver your hard-to-find healthcare products to your door!
See ad page 105

8578 Santa Monica Blvd./4454 Van Nuys Blvd.

West Hollywood   *(310) 289-1125*
Sherman Oaks   *(818) 905-8338*
    (800) 819-9098

Health Pharm

The best of nutritional supplements, homeopathic remedies, herbs, pure bath products, synergy, colloidal silver, and essential oils. See ad page 81
128 Old Topanga Canyon Rd.
Topanga, CA   90290

(310) 455-3370

Merit Homeopathy

We carry Homeopathics, Herbs, Vitamins, Colloidals, Essential Oils, Flower Essences, Progest, Ear Cones and Chlorad.
See ad page 106
Knollwood Pharmacy, 11862 Balboa Blvd.
Granada Hills, CA   91344

(818) 831-1727

Phoenix Wellness Center

A True Wellness Center which blends Eastern and Western medicine in complete harmony. Herbs, aromatherapy, acupuncture, homeopathics, essential oils, bulk herbs and teas. See ad page 112
2515-2523 East Washington Blvd.
Pasadena, CA   91104.

(626) 791-7600 or (626) 398-5400

Santa Monica Homeopathic Pharmacy

Family owned and operated pharmacy specializing in healthy alternatives, including homeopathics, herbs, Chinese herbs, nutritional supplements, aromatherapy and health & beauty products. Knowledge, care and service since 1944. See ad page 94
629 Broadway, Santa Monica, CA   90401

(310) 395-7861   (310) 395-1131 FAX

S & J Pharmacy

Homeopathic and Herbal Pharmacy:
Ayurvedic formulas, homeopathic remedies,
vitamins, magnets, and nutritional
supplements. Consultations with herbalist,
John Kulak, O.M.D. See ad page 114

8415 Reseda Blvd. Suite 6
Northridge, CA   91324

(818) 700-2956 or (818) 700-0513

Warner Plaza Pharmacy

Homeopathics, prescriptions, books,
vitamins, herbs, and sports nutrition.
Acupuncture, Steven Shaw, LAc.
See ad page 73

21733 Ventura Blvd.
Woodland Hills, CA   91364.

(818) 348-0524

Expect nothing. Live frugally
On surprise.

—ALICE WALKER

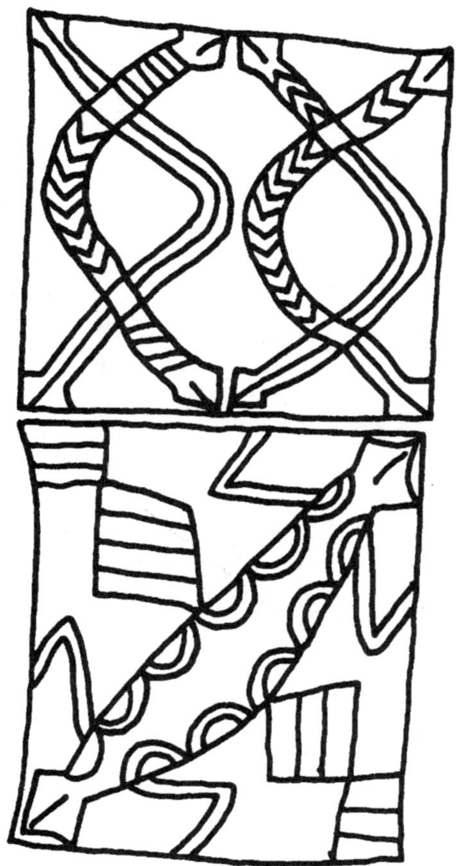

HOLISTIC PHYSICIANS PRACTITIONERS

*H*olistic practitioners of traditional Eastern and Western methods view a person's body, mind and spirit as integral to health and healing. They consider, rather than just the disease and its symptoms, the physical, nutritional, emotional, environmental and spiritual levels. They also seek non-invasive alternatives. Holistic practitioners develop cooperative relationships with fellow practitioners of complementary modalities. They also encourage their clients to take an active role in their healing process.

Continued

Acupuncture, part of Traditional Chinese Medicine, has been practiced for over 3,500 years in China. It is based on the belief that 'chi' energy circulates throughout the body along specific pathways called meridians. The blocking of energy in the meridians due to physiological imbalances, results in stress, pain and disease. Practitioners insert fine, disposable, sterile needles into the surface of the skin at specific points along the meridians to re-establish the flow of 'chi' and promote the body's own natural healing ability.

Jacklin Arastouzadeh
L.Ac., Lipl.Ac. Dipl. NBAO

Licensed Acupuncturist and Chinese herbalist. Diplomat of Orthopedics, Research acupuncturist, UCLA Medical Center. See ad page 79

462 N. Linden Dr. Ste. 336
Beverly Hills, CA 90212

(310) 777-0388

Marcy J. Basel, L.Ac., Dipl.Ac NCCA

Traditional Acupuncture and herbal medicine specializing in chronic pain, digestive disorders and female problems, returning the body to its natural state of balance. See ad page 86

Santa Monica

(310) 829-1233

Mindy Boxer, Ph.D., L.Ac., Dipl.Ac.,D.Hom.

Naturoprathic Medicine treats the whole person with natural therapies to stimulate your body's innate healing capacities. *Acupuncture & Chinese Herbs:* Ancient Medicine healing the Modern World. See ad page 109

3301 Ocean Park Blvd. Suite 201
Santa Monica, CA   90405

(310) 450-9711

Marsha Connor, L.Ac., OMD, RN

Complete holistic approach combining Oriental and Western medicine. Effective and safe techniques for children are utilized.

Mount Washington   *(323) 225-0820*

Eileen Hamsa Henry, L.Ac., O.M.D.

A Doctor of Oriental Medicine with a holistic approach devoted to individual personalized health care. Dr. Henry employs state of the art diagnostic methods to uncover the root of chronic illness. See ad page 90

Brentwood Center for Wellness
11611 San Vicente Blvd.
Los Angeles, CA. 90049

(310) 826-8606) (310) 826-8446 FAX

Dr. Roger C. Hirsh, OMD, L.Ac.

Traditional Oriental Medicine, Acupuncture, Herbal Medicine and Qi Kung Therapy. Specializing in the Reproductive Healthcare needs for Healthy couples to have Healthy children. We at Metamedical Group feel there are many types of health challenges that can be helped by Oriental medicine. Practicing since 1974. See ad page 76

RHIRSH@METAMED.COM

9730 Wilshire Blvd. Suite 105
Beverly Hills, CA   90212

(310) 550-8186

Institute for Health,
Teresa Rispoli, L.Ac., Ph.D.

Acupuncture is a complete medical system used to diagnose and prevent illness and improve well-being as well as eliminate pain. See ad page 99

28247 Agoura Rd.
Agoura Hills, CA   91301

(818) 707-3126 (818) 707-2787 FAX

Lakshmi Lambert, L.Ac., Dipl.Ac.
Family Health Center

Respectful Health Care in an intimate setting. Sessions are one-to-one for $1\frac{1}{2}$ hours. 8 years as a licensed Acupuncture Physician. 18 years as an Herbalist. 13 years as a Bodyworker. Background as a psychotherapist. I specialize in Pediatrics, Women's Health, Emotional Health and Pain Management. Emphasis on Patient education and transformation. Improved health and well-being after one session.

Westside　　　　　　　**(310) 737-1998**

Flo with Health

Flo Lawrence, L.Ac., D.O.M., B.S. (Ed.), M.S. (Ed.)
Through Acupuncture/Herbs and Massage Therapy, I help relieve pain, balance energies, build immunities and prevent and care for disease. See ad page 91

Topanga & Los Angeles

　　(310) 455-2857　(310) 455-3197 FAX

Nancy Marcucella, D.C., LAc.

Acupuncture, Bodywork, Chiropractic. Building blocks to health. See ad page 77
email: topabc@webtv.net
Call for free consultation.
131 South Topanga Canyon Blvd.
Topanga, CA 90290

　　(310) 455-3577　(310) 455-0860 FAX

Radiant Health

Michael J. Maguire, L.Ac.
Acupuncture. Herbal Medicine. Nutrition. Specializing in individualized programs for anti-aging, gynecology and pediatric nutrition. Expert in recurrent ear infections, hair mineral analysis, lymphatic detox therapy, and soft tissue restructuring. Chi Kung classes. See ad page 96
radhealth@earthlink.net
4003 Michael Ave, L.A., CA 90066

　　　　(310) 306-4771 or (888) 220-4153
Malibu　　　　　　**(310) 457-4714 FAX**

Spirit's Flight Healing Arts

Laura Paris, O.M.D., L.Ac.
Over 12 years experience in Oriental and Energetic Healing Arts, Herbs and Homeopathy. Spiritual Acupuncture and Spirit's Flight ancient Absuchan Ka Healings designed to elevate the spirit. See ad page 78
1502 Montana Ave. Ste.202, S.M., CA 90403

　　　　(310) 458-7738 or (800) 605-9555

Karen L. Raub, N.D., L.Ac.

Regain control of your health. Find safe alternatives to surgery. Reduce drug side effects. Prevent recurring health problems. Herbal consultation and acupuncture available by appointment. See ad page 97

Pasadena　　　　　　**(626) 391-5419**

Michael Sax, L.Ac.

Licensed Acupuncturist. Diplomate of Chinese Herbology. Nutrition and lifestyle counseling, women's health issues, chronic physical pain, emotional/mental pattern release, natural weight loss, internal cleansing and detoxification, stress and depression, addictions and chemical dependency.

Santa Monica　　　　　**(310) 393-6642**
Redondo Beach　　　　**(310) 540-0163**

Patricia Walton, L.Ac., Dipl.Ac.

Acupuncture, Acupressure and Herbology.

Santa Monica　　　　　**(310) 453-0286**

CHIROPRACTIC

The practice of spinal manipulation has been used since at least the 5th century B.C. "Chiropractic" was developed by Canadian, David D. Palmer in 1895. It corrects nerve interference in the body primarily through the use of hands-on manipulation of the spine, joints and muscles. Adjustment of misaligned vertebrae relieves pressure on nerve roots within the spinal column, maintaining the health of the central nervous system and organs. The body's inherent ability to heal itself is then able to work to maximum efficiency.

Continued

Essential Chiropractic Center
David Bond D.C., QME, D.J.Hom.

Spinal manipulation, non-force, gentle chiropractic, deep tissue release therapy. Family, pregnancy and child care. Exercise and nutritional counseling. Athletic, personal and work injury. See ad page 107
15720 Ventura Blvd. Suite 101B
Encino, CA 91436   **(818) 501-8743**

Durgin Chiropractic & Naturopathic Clinic

Chiropractic: gentle but effective chiropractic that incorporates Naturopathic manipulative techniques from pediatric to geriatric. See ad page 125
612 Santa Monica Blvd., Santa Monica, CA 90401
(310) 576-6176

Dean Goodman
Chiropractor and Health Educator

Gentle, effective, hands-on chiropractic care relieves pain and awakens the self-healing capacity of your body. Alignment of body, mind and spirit restores health and helps you fulfill your potential. With 17 years of experience, Dr. Goodman is post-graduate faculty at Cleveland Chiropractic College and is currently President of the Santa Monica Chiropractic Society.
720 Wilshire Blvd. #210, Santa Monica, CA 90401
(310) 395-5504

Kerry Hill D.C.

Family Chiropractic and Nutrition: I use gentle and non-force chiropractic techniques to treat families, including children and pregnant women. I also use state of the art assessments to design individual nutritional and lifestyle programs for optimum health including infant nutrition. See ad page 103
Santa Monica   **(310) 458-0400**

Donald C. Kelliher, D.C.

We practice chiropractic with an emphasis on the complete person, specializing in chronic conditions. We revitalize normal biochemical function and revive uninterrupted nerve flow to the tissues. Full health restored.
Malibu, Agoura & Beverly Hills
(310) 457-2047   (818) 707-6006

Dr. Stephanie M. King
Chiropractic Physician

Personalized Alternative Health Care for Families. Chiropractic Biophysics Analysis for Total Body Wellness. Nutritional Counseling and Herbal Supplementation. Specializing in Sports Injuries and Rehabilitation for Athletes. See ad page 79
San Marino   **(626) 799-0557**

Phina McBride D.C.

Dr. Phina McBride brings to her clients experience in not only chiropractic work but sacro-occipital therapy, craniopathy and intuitive diagnosis. She joins her gifts as a healer with Kenton Lane, psychic astrologer, and Camille Tyler, tarot, in the Entrada Healing Group. See ad page 108
1328 Westwood Blvd., Ste. 9 L.A., CA 90024
(310) 441-9311

Network Spinal Analysis of Los Angeles
Ruth Ziemba, D.C., R.N., C.M.T.

"Begin the journey to vibrant health." A unique, gentle and powerful method. Network Spinal Analysis is a life-enhancing form of Chiropractic that uses a network of techniques timed for when the body can best receive them. Network Spinal Analysis improves health and well-being while raising your capacity to deal better with life stresses.See ad page 122
1026 S. Robertson Blvd. Ste.300, L.A., CA 90035
(310) 657-2352   (310) 358-0978 FAX

Ptak Chiropractic Life Center

Ptak Chiropractic Life Center is dedicated to optimal wellness and the fulfillment of one's maximum potential as a human

being. Spinal cord and spinal nerve stress interfere with our ability to express life to its maximum. With computerized technology, we can objectively test for the presence or absence of spinal nerve stress. You are never too young or too old to live free of spinal nerve stress.
healthptak@earthlink.net
1127 Wilshire Blvd. Santa Monica

(310) 451-5336

Total Body Wellness Center

Dr. Steven I. Sherwin

Feel your body function in complete balance. We assist you in removing interferences to your nervous system, utilizing a variety of approaches: neuroemotional techniques to nurture your soul; herbal supplements and homeopathic remedies to detoxify and strengthen your body; and chiropractics to align your system for full potential. Progress monitored with a SEMG system...a painless, non-invasive test, characterizing abnormal activity of muscles surrounding the spine. Call for a new experience in health care.

See ad page 92
22601 Pacific Coast Hwy., Suite 225
Malibu, CA 90265   **(310) 456-3427**

Catherine Veritas D.C.

Holistic Chiropractic - from subtle energy balance to orthopedic injury rehabilitation.
West Los Angeles   **(310) 826-3385**
Topanga   **(310) 455-1152**

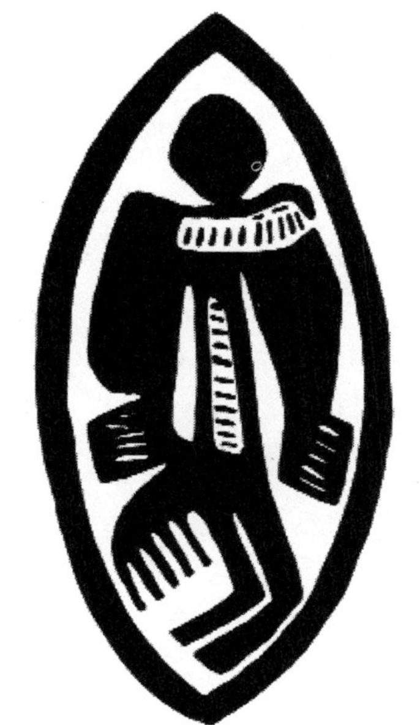

—OSCAR WILDE

Homeopathy, based on the Law of Similars, is a healing principle proposing that natural substances, which can cause disease when given in large doses, promote healing when given in micro doses. These natural substances stimulate and remove toxins from the body, allowing a person to regain balance and health.

Flower essences focus on healing the emotional body during times of crises and stress, while herbology uses whole plants and creates 'synergistic' formulas with therapeutic effects treating particular viral and infectious illnesses.

Anne W. Dupuis
Consultant/ Educator
English Flower Essences in the Tradition of Dr. Edward Bach.
Santa Monica   **(310) 393-3865**

Lauren S. Feder, M.D.
Homeopathy is a healing process which encourages the body's natural healing forces of recovery. Dr. Feder treats children, adults and conditions during pregnancy and breastfeeding. Also, ongoing natural parenting and childbirth workshops. See ad page 74
415 N. Crescent Dr., Suite 100
Beverly Hills, CA 90210
(310) 247-1531

Merit Homeopathy
Remedies available in Tincture, Pellets, Tablets, X & C Potencies, Combinations, Ointment and Creams. See ad page 106
Knollwood Pharmacy
11862 Balboa Blvd.
Granada Hills, CA 91344
(818) 831-1727

Monastery of Herbs
Michael George Philips, Ph.D. & Assoc.
27 years specializing in Bacteria, Viruses, Fungi, and Parasites. From a Monastic setting we manufacture "custom designed" Herbal Blends. Immune system re-structuring is our specialty. Private formulations for practitioners are available. See ad page 119
L.A., Valley & Global   **(818) 360-4871**

Spirit's Flight Healing Arts
Laura Paris, O.M.D., L.Ac.
Oriental and Energetic Healing Arts, Herbs and Homeopathy. Spiritual Acupuncture treatments designed to move consciousness to a higher level. Spirit's Flight ancient Absuchan Ka Healings designed to elevate the soul. See ad page 78
1502 Montana Ave. Suite 202
Santa Monica, CA 90403
(310) 458-7738
(800) 605-9555

Jeffrey Garson Shapiro, HD, Ph.D.
Homeopathy, Flower Essences, Holistic Health & Nutrition. See ad page 103
Santa Monica   **(310) 458-6099**

"Twilight is the crack between the worlds."
—CARLOS CASTANEDA

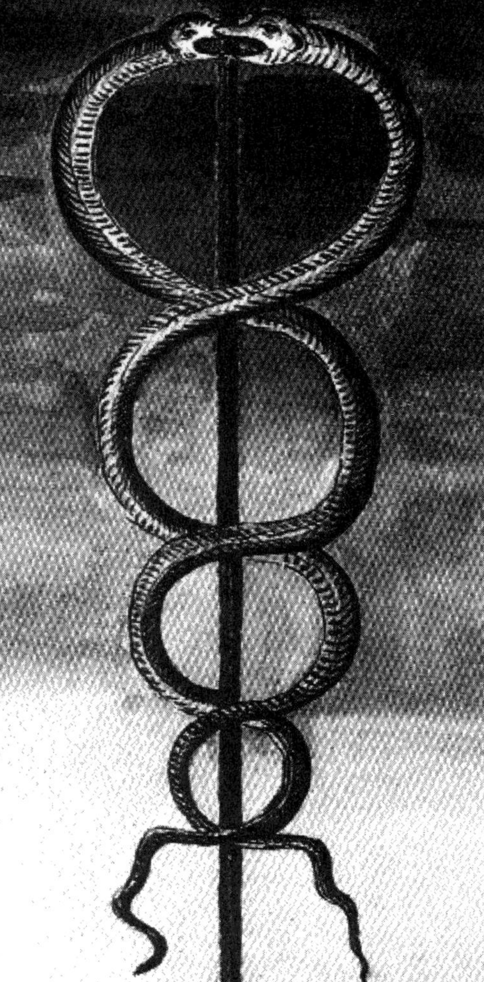

HYPNOTHERAPY

Hypnotherapy puts the conscious mind in a trance state, allowing access to the highly suggestible subconscious. This modality facilitates personal growth through the release of blocks due to forgotten or suppressed memories and through the correction of negative beliefs or habits. Treatments may focus on relieving simple addictions or sourcing core issues that create imbalances.

Monika Grill

A wholistic Therapy Program utilizing metaphysical principles and mental, emotional and energetic tools for empowerment. See ad page 107

West Los Angeles   **(310) 207-0675**

Lane LaRue & Joe Futterer Certified Hypnotherapists

Change Your Life with Hypnosis. Stop smoking. Erase fear of flying. Improve study and test results. Reduce and control pain. Enhance physical therapy. Reduce anxiety and stress. Control anger. Improve sports performance. Be more successful. Topanga & San Fernando Valley

(818) 704-7011

IRIDOLOGY

The eye's iris includes thousands of nerve endings linked to every body organ and tissue. To the trained practitioner, the iris can reveal illness, degeneration and inherent weaknesses in the body. For example, toxic conditions, organ weaknesses, and your medical history can all be diagnosed through the eyes. Psychological conditions can also be pinpointed. Holistic physicians may use iridology as a diagnostic tool in the treatment of their clients.

Institute for Health

Teresa Rispoli, L.Ac., Ph.D.

The eyes possess a map to the various body systems and organs and can disclose varying degrees of ill health and inherent weaknesses in the body. See ad page 99

28247 Agoura Rd.
Agoura Hills, CA   91301

(818) 707-3126   (818) 707-2787 FAX

Holistic Medical Doctors practice integrated medicine. Unlike specialists who focus intently and become expert in one particular field, holistic doctors are aware of the overall make up of an individual. They employ not only standard medical procedures, but also holistic practices such as acupuncture, herbal remedies, nutritionist and homeopathic cures. Rather than imposing the same prescription on everyone with similar symptoms, they tend to act more in partnership with you to find the best technique for your healing process.

Lauren S. Feder, M.D.

Homeopathy is a healing process which encourages the body's natural healing forces of recovery. Dr. Feder treats children, adults and conditions during pregnancy and breastfeeding. Also, ongoing natural parenting and childbirth workshops. See ad page 74
415 N. Crescent Dr., Suite 100
Beverly Hills, CA 90210

(310) 247-1531

Steven M. Krems, M.D.

Board Certified Internal Medicine. Herbal medicine, acupuncture, In-office body-work. The best of integrative medicine.
4644 Lincoln Blvd., Suite 111
Marina Del Rey   (310) 306-6966

Gayle Madeleine Randall, M.D.

Integrative practitioner with extensive scientific knowledge and unique experience with ancient healing and spirituality. She embraces the powerful combination of different medicines because "true healing occurs through balancing of all planes - physical, emotional, mental and spiritual."
Malibu   (310) 456-9393

Shera Raisen, M.D.

Shera Raisen, M.D. is a western trained physician who integrates alternative therapies to attain optimal health and treat diseases, such as digestive disorders, fatigue and menopause. She enjoys women's health, gynecology and preventative care. See ad page 72
900 Wilshire Blvd. Suite 450
Santa Monica CA 90403

(310) 394-7277 (310) 394-7147 FAX

Born from Hippocrates and later "nature cures" in 19th century spa towns of Austria and Germany, Naturopathy believes the body's natural state is one of equilibrium, which can be upset by an unhealthy lifestyle. Naturopathic Doctors emphasize prevention and use natural remedies and therapies to promote the body's inherent healing powers. They carefully select non-invasive remedies that have the least side effects. Naturopaths often work in conjunction with medical doctors and specialists to provide patients with holistic treatment options.

Aesculapius

Naturopathic Medical Clinic's Specialties: lifestyle counseling and psychotherapy, herbology, nutrition and kineseology.
1111 Topanga Canyon Blvd. Suite 6
Topanga, CA   90290

(310) 455-2282

Durgin Chiropractic & Naturopathic Clinic

Naturopathic: Bastyr graduate with 15 years of practice experience. Focus on nutrition, herbs, female conditions, cancer. See ad page 125

612 Santa Monica Blvd.
Santa Monica, CA   90401

(310) 576-6176

Health Integration Center

Rex Wilson, Naturopath

I am a graduate of National College of Naturopathic Medicine and have over 20 years of clinical experience. Along with my Naturopathic services, our center offers traditional and holistic medicine, acupuncture, lymphatic therapy and Hellerwork. Balancing body chemistry, optimizing energy and immunity, and helping you to fulfill your optimum health potential is our goal. Find out how you can benefit from homeopathy, herbal remedies, right diet and nutritional support, electrodermal screening and other advances in natural healthcare by calling for a free information packet.

1431 7th St. Suite 201
Santa Monica, CA 90401

(310) 656-7978

Karen L. Raub, N.D., L.Ac.

Regain control of your health. Find safe alternatives to surgery. Reduce drug side effects. Prevent recurring health problems. Herbal consultation and acupuncture available by appointment. See ad page 97

Pasadena   **(626) 791-7600**

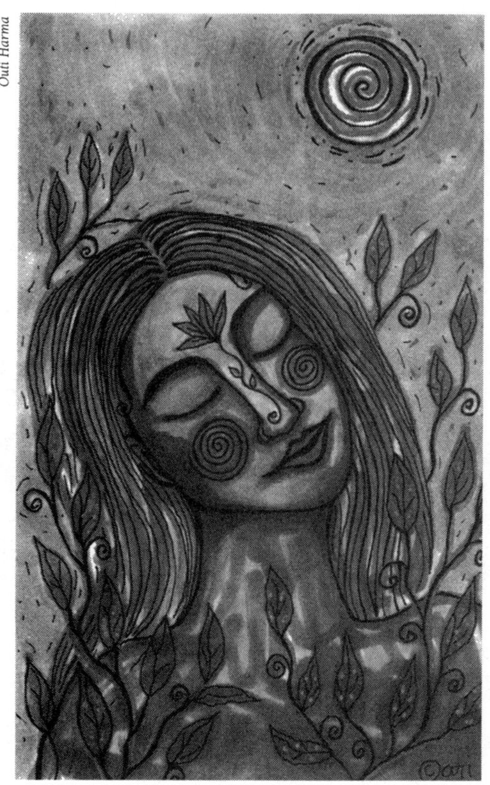

... such stuff
As dreams are made on ...
—WILLIAM SHAKESPEARE

HOLISTIC WELLWOMAN PRE & POST NATAL CARE

Holistic Wellwoman centers and pre and post natal services provide care for women by women. These caregivers use non-invasive techniques to assist and support all aspects of women's health and all phases of this life giving process.

Judy Bravard, CNP, Nurse Practitioner
Pacifica Women's Health Care
11101 Venice Blvd.
Los Angeles, CA   90034   *(310) 840-5755*

Natural Birth and Women's Center
Women's healthcare, Gynecology, PMS counseling, Infertility counseling, Menopause, Nutritional consulting, Comprehensive pre-natal care. See ad page 93
14140 Magnolia Blvd.
Sherman Oaks, CA 91423

(818) 386-1082

Luciann Rosen, R.N.,M.N.,C-F.N.P.
Breast Care, herbology, nutrition and spiritual healing.
Santa Monica Bay Physicians
804 7th St., Santa Monica, CA 90403
(310)395-5588

A doula, from the Greek meaning "mothering the mother" or "woman caregiver," supports a pregnant woman and her partner either pre and post natally in the home or during labor at home births, in birth centers or hospitals.

Dayo Doula Care
Kari Hopson, Founder
Pre and post partum care. Birth services. 24 hour service available. Established 1989.
(310) 236-6043

Cordelia Hanna, Certified Childbirth Educator, Certified Birth Assistant
Full Childbirth Support Services: Wholistic Childbirth Education & Labor Support. Prepare for natural childbirth at home, in hospital or birth center while cultivating acceptance of unexpected outcomes.
http://home.earthlink.net/~shehina/
shehina@earthlink.net
Los Angeles County   *(626) 358-2318*

Davi K. Khalsa, R.N., CCE
Childbirth Education Classes and labor support: The most complete up to date techniques and information available.
Los Angeles   *(310) 273-2385*

A Mother's Touch
PreNatal Massage & Doula Care Service: Our postpartum doulas provide nurturing care and support to new mothers, babies and families. Services include: breastfeeding support, well baby care instruction, natural comfort measures, nutritious meal

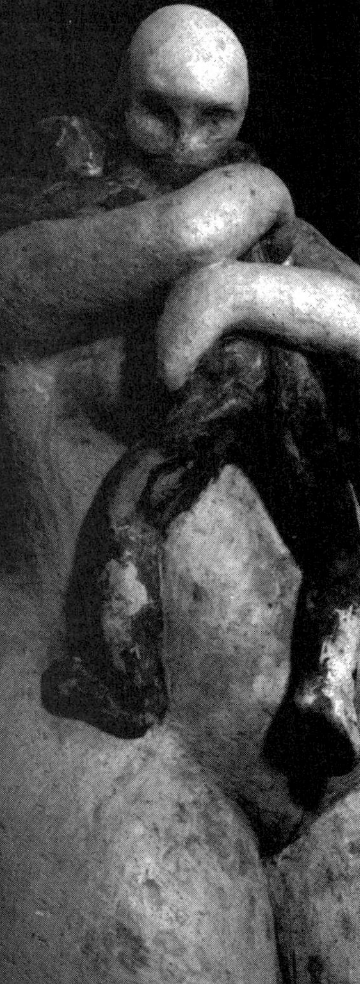

preparation and practical household assistance. Prenatal and postpartum relaxation massage sessions are available in the comfort of your home.

Los Angeles — (888) 644-9595

Tracy Hartley & Carmen Bornn-Gilman

Birth Doula services throughout the greater Los Angeles area. See ad page 124
Doulatracy@AOL.com
http://members.AOL.com/Doulatracy/index.html

(626) 284-0447 or (818) 507-5785

Claudia Udy

Bringing together father and mother for a quality birthing experience and intimate support for the single parent.

Topanga and Westside — (310) 455-7026

INFANT/PREGNANCY MASSAGE/YOGA

Specially trained massage practitioners focus on relief of lower back pain, leg swelling, soreness and fatigue. This practice increases circulation, normalizes sleep patterns and enhances a sense of well-being for mothers. Infants benefit from sensory awareness, release of tension and circulatory stimulation.

Amanda Bailey

Pre-natal & post natal massage. Experienced in high risk pregnancy and bed risk, pregnancy cushions. Insurance accepted.

Westside — (310) 822-4504

Elyse Briggs
Licensed Massage Therapist

Specializing in Prenatal, Thai, Swedish, Deep Tissue and Profound Relaxation. See ad page 104
ak413@latn.org
BRIGGSBODYWORKS@www.geocities.com/HOTSPRINGS/SPA/8162/

Glendale — (818) 241-1781

Marla Mattenson, L.M.T.

Learn how to nurture your baby through unconditional loving touch the way only a parent can. As a licensed massage therapist, I will give you the specific techniques you need to deepen the bond and enhance what you already know with your baby. Group and private classes; Doctor recommended.

Santa Monica & Los Angeles

(310) 588-1187

Caitlin Philips, Ms.T., CD

Offers a wide variety of body/mind techniques from Eastern to Western, including pre-natal & childbirth assistance.

Office located at West Los Angeles/ Santa Monica border.

(310) 239-4023

Yoga Baby Studio

Specializing in pre-natal, labor preparation, Baby and Me. Also Hatha, Ashtanga and privates. Call Rocki.

Venice   *(310) 306-9381*

MIDWIFERY

Midwives attend women during the childbirth process in a variety of settings and are trained to care for women before, during, after and between pregnancies. Well trained in all aspects of the birthing process, they always provide back up scenarios in case of unforeseen complications. Worldwide, eighty percent of all babies are received into the skilled, caring hands of midwives, and according to the Center of Disease Control, home births with midwives are the safest birthing practices in the United States.

Shelly Girard

Childbirth at Home - A Labor of Love. Wholistic Midwifery and Well-Woman Gynecological Care.

anahata@earthlink.net   www.socalbirth.org

Los Angeles   *(323) 221-7822*

Home Birth Service of Los Angeles

Felicia Forrest, CNM, Leslie Stewart, CNM

Prenatal care, home births and well woman health care by midwives.

3959 Laurel Canyon Blvd. Suite A
Studio City, CA   91604

                      (818) 760-6541

Nancy Marshutz

Natural Childbirth Institute

Full-scope nurse mid-wifery practice. We take care of pre-natal, delivery, and post-partum needs of well women. We do underwater births and family planning.
nanbaby@earthlink.net

4260 Beverly Blvd.
Los Angeles   **(323) 462-8682**

Meadow Born for Pure Birthing

Lani Rose Jeansdottir, CPM, LM, MA

Midwifery services. Home birth. Well-woman gynecology. Cervical caps. Mother to be and Baby blessings.
See ad page 124
meadowborn@geocities.com
http://www.geocities.com/wellesley/2713

                      (818) 347-1493

Westside Birth Service

Louana Seibold, RN, PHN

Discover the holism of midwifery care and home birth.

2442 Euclid St. Santa Monica, CA 90405

                      (310) 452-3020

Louanne Watson, MSN, CNM

Homebirths With Louanne. Certified Nurse Midwife. Homebirth practice; Christian nurse-midwife with 14 years of experience.
homecnm@aol.com

San Gabriel   *(626) 256-4663*

NATURAL FERTILITY METHODS

Doctors and practitioners look for natural methods to enhance your system's ability to function at optimum levels. Without resorting to expensive drug therapies, practitioners pinpoint ovulation cycles and stimulate production of healthy eggs and sperm. Practitioners assist you through to successful conception.

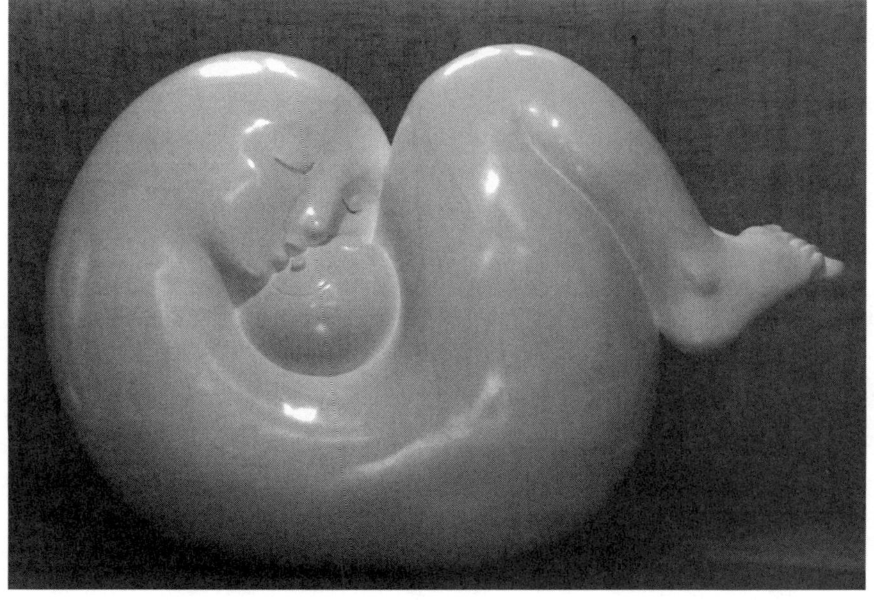

Megan Rice

Soul is the poetry of our lives...
—Thomas Moore

HYDROTHERAPEUTIC COLONICS

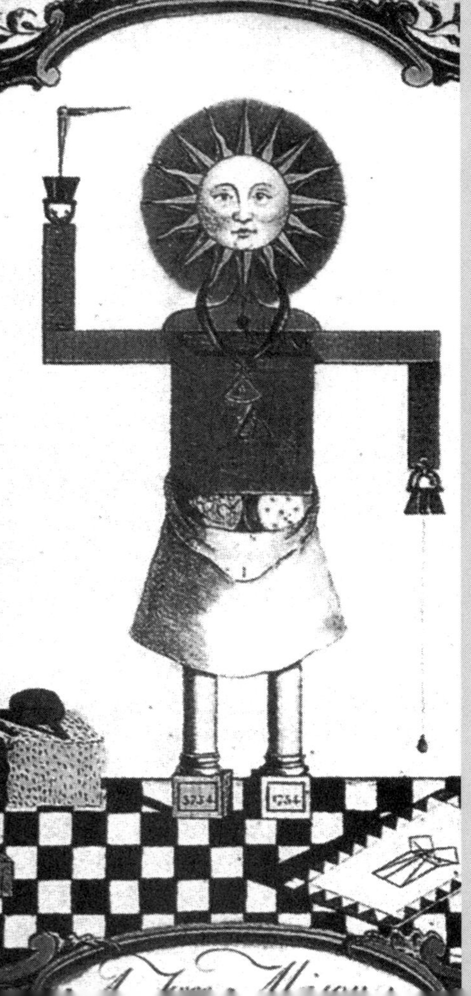

Hydrotherapeutic Colonics gently cleanses the colon, allowing the body to detoxify from modern day pollutants and poor dietary habits. Conditions that colon therapy helps include: allergies, anxiety, backaches, colitis, constipation, fatigue, headaches, hemorrhoids, indigestion, toxemia, and water retention.

BodyZAlive

BodyZAlive offers a safe, discreet, holistic environment with state-of-the-art equipment, disposable attachments and purified water for gentle cleansing colon hydrotherapy. BodyZAlive also offers seaweed and herbal body wraps. See ad page 123

1137 2nd St. Suite 205
Santa Monica, CA   90403

(310) 587-2639

Institute for Health

Teresa Rispoli, L.Ac., Ph.D.

Colonics cleanse the bowel and blood, empower the immune system, restore pH balance, and rejuvenate every cell in the body. See ad page 99

28247 Agoura Rd.
Agoura Hills, CA 91301

(818) 707-3126   (818) 707-2787 FAX

Ventura Center for Healing

Holistic Healing Center in the San Fernando Valley offering: Colon Hydrotherapy, Therapeutic Massage, Detoxifying Body Wraps, Nutrition with Herbs & Diet, Foot Reflexology, and Air & Water Purification Systems.

19525 Ventura Blvd.
Tarzana, CA 91356

(818) 343-3571   (818) 343-0224 FAX

MARTIAL ARTS

Conscious awareness of our body, breath, mind and soul is inherent in the practice of martial arts such as T'ai Chi, Qi Gong, Karate and Kun Tao. Exercises focus the whole being in fluid and/or sharp motion. Alignment and subtle connection with energies of all nature's kingdoms awaken us to being 'completely present' with increased alertness, physical stamina and relaxation.

Mathew Cohen

Explore the world of internal and external martial arts from China and Indonesia. Kun Tao Silat is a blend of traditional and progressive reality based trainings for self defense, spiritual expression and health. Twenty years in Martial Arts, Dance and other body-mind disciplines. Mathew has a Martial Arts and Massage practice in Santa Monica and teaches internationally. See ad page 77

Santa Monica   **(310) 392-6788**

Theresa Hoff

Instruction for the internal healing arts of Tai Chi and Qi Gong. Integration of breathing exercises, Aura-Soma therapy and meditation.

231 Vista Del Mar Suite C
Redondo Beach, CA   90277

(310) 834-2361

Montgomery Karate

"If there's no enemy within, the enemy without can do us no harm." —*African proverb.* "There is nothing that I can do something about, if it's nothing but to adjust myself to an unpleasant situation so that it doesn't destroy my spirit. I am here to tell you that if you are seeking a goal, being successful in reaching that goal will require all of the discipline that one can muster from within their body." —*Napolean Hill.* Children, Women and Men.
See ad page 127

Topanga/Los Angeles   **(310) 455-9557**

Lana Spraker

Peaceful Way T'ai Chi Ch'uan

26 years teaching Traditional Yang style & Qi Gong. See ad page 93

West Los Angeles & Santa Monica

(310) 479-3646

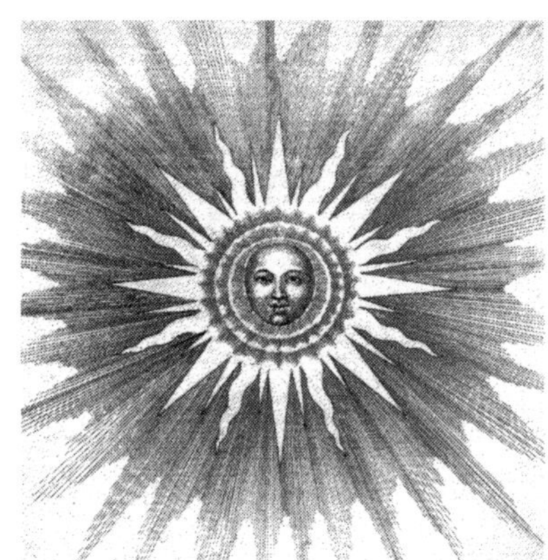

"Our Dreams are our real life"
—Frederico Fellini

MASSAGE AND BODY-MIND THERAPIES

Massage and Body-Mind Therapies honor the integrity of mind-body-spirit wholeness in individuals. Drawing on Eastern and Western disciplines, practitioners support their clients in restoring union and balance within themselves through structural, fluid, muscular, central nervous, organ, emotional and/or energetic systems.

Craniosacral therapy claims that the cranial 'rhythmic impulse' affects every cell in the body. Expanding on cranial osteopathy which massages the bones of our head, craniosacral practitioners massage the membranes encasing the brain and spinal cord to restore the complete functioning of the craniosacral system. This practice corrects imbalances in the central nervous system between the cranium and the sacrum, resetting the body's natural healing potential.

Marcy J. Basel, L.Ac., CSI, CSII, SERI
Visceral Manipulation
CranioSacral therapy encourages natural healing for the central nervous system through light touch hands-on therapy. See ad page 86

Santa Monica (310) 829-1233

Tracy Griffiths
Craniosacral therapy is a healing art that helps you get related to the self-correcting ebb and flow of your Craniosacral system, the cranial bones, spine and sacrum, your spinal fluid and your entire connective tissue system. This enhances your own healing ability and process. See ad page 95

Topanga (310) 455-9381

Institute for Health
Teresa Rispoli, L.Ac., Ph.D.
Craniosacral therapy encourages your system to dissipate the negative effects of stress and enhance general health and resistance to disease, utilizing the therapist's light hands-on approach. See ad page 99
28247 Agoura Rd.
Agoura Hills, CA   91301

(818) 707-3126   (818) 707-2787 FAX

Gloria Kamler, M.A.
Practical, holistic educator. Gifted hands, 25 years experience. Specializing in: Polarity stress release, Lymphatic detox, Cranio-sacral trauma resolution.
See ad page 85
Santa Monica School of Integrated Studies
Santa Monica (310) 450-4541

"To see a world in a grain of sand and heaven in a wildflower; Hold infinity in the palm of your hand And eternity in an hour."
—WILLIAM BLAKE

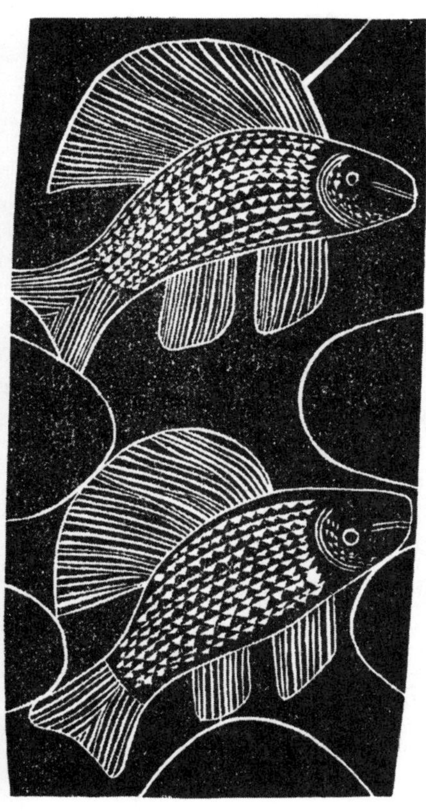

Whether named energy, prana, life force, or 'chi,' cultures around the world acknowledge energy as a source of life. Through body-mind techniques, practitioners touch the energies within and surrounding individuals with intentions of clearing and balancing. By incorporating physical practices, practitioners also align the body, allowing energy to flow freely. Clear, balanced, flowing energy succeeds in harmonizing the body, mind and soul.

Creative Light Workers

Trine Richter & Alan Clancy

Reiki Masters and Teachers. Intuitive, guided journeys and Shiatsu. Allow yourself to trust and activate your own guidance.

Santa Monica (Trine)   *(310) 314-2262*
Hollywood (Alan)   *(213) 212-5269*

Diane Dalbey, M.A., CST, CMT
Lighten Up

Relieve physical and emotional traumas; increase energy and balance with BodyMind therapies such as CranioSacral, medical Qigong, Psychological Anatomy, humor and dialogue techniques. Gentle and respectful.
See ad page 115
LYGHTNUP@AOL.COM

Sherman Oaks   *(818) 501-4280*

Tony Franco, Ms.T., M.A.

The compassionate heart of holistic healing through wellness-affirming psychospiritual bioenergetics. Counseling psychology, craniosacral therapy, spiritual healing, aromatherapy and massage.

Culver City   *(310) 390-2528*

Linda S. Garrett

Achieve Inner Peace: Experience the unique qualities of body harmony & Reiki. The non-intrusive techniques employ a butterfly-like touch while creating a calm & safe space, allowing body, mind, spirit & emotions to meld & evolve. Also practicing flower essence therapy. Reiki Master.
nrpcelsg@aol.com

Encino   *(818) 981-3522*

Leeta Kunnel

Transformational bodywork. Energy balancing. Movement and sound therapy. Assisting harmonious flow and relationship with your body, mind and spirit.
See ad page 119

                            (310) 281-9787

Rosanne Mangio

Works in the following modalities:
Vibrational Healing, Massage Therapy,
Fluid Body Coaching, Essential Oil
Therapy, Footbone Massage and Reiki.
See ad page 82

(310) 459-3044

Karl Schleinig

Energy Healer, Bodyworker, Meditation
Teacher: Heart-Centered Energy healing
to assist you in accepting, transmitting
and integrating blocked energies. The
anchoring of spiritual energies in the subtle
and physical bodies opens us to more
awareness, compassion and healthy living.
By appointment or in home.
Marina del Rey   (310) 821-6103

Amy Thakurdas, L.L.M., B.A.

Sounds of Light: Gentle energetic cleansing
and balancing of the physical and subtle
bodies, using sound, color, crystals, aromatherapy and energetic touch. A
variety of holistic principles including Chi
Gong, Reiki, herbs and past life regression
are offered. See ad page 80
Los Angeles   (323) 874-3096

Pamela Ann Wheeler

Holistic Facilitator. *Comfort Zone*. Magnetic
Energy Balancing. See ad page 80
healthzone@aol.com
La Canada/Pasadena

(818) 790-9278   (818) 790-5181 FAX

HELLERWORK

*Hellerwork is a dynamic system integrating
structural bodywork and movement
re-education with an opportunity to explore
how stress, habits and emotions impact the
body and influence one's health and
well-being.*

Carol Bretonne

Wellness through deep tissue bodywork,
movement education, guided dialogue.
Member of Assoc. Bodywork & Massage
Professionals.
Malibu & Pacific Palisades

(310) 457-4863

Mari Hotaki

I work with comforting and relieving all
levels of pain. Specializing in pre and post
natal care.
1514 17th St., Suite 203
Santa Monica, CA 90403

(310) 394-7909

Rita Kathlyn

Certified Hellerwork Practitioner
Movement education, craniosacral therapy,
sports injury, and massage therapy.
Topanga & Westside   (310) 455-3615

Helene Zuckerman

Certified Hellerwork Practitioner
Along with physical changes of improved
posture, increased flexibility and vitality,
and relief from chronic tension and pain,
Helene teaches people to listen and
respond to the wisdom that lives in their
bodies. As people learn the particular
language of their body, it becomes an ally
in living life from the heart.
Ohana Healing Arts
1514 17th St. #203,
Santa Monica, CA 90404

(310) 453-0286

LYMPHATIC MASSAGE

*The lymph system, part of the immune
system, affects the entire body. Excess
toxins, pollutants, viruses, bacteria
and other waste materials in the body
accumulate in the lymph nodes, causing
them to swell and become painful. Lymph
massage improves drainage of the nodes
and circulation of the fluids.*

Institute for Health

Teresa Rispoli, L.Ac., Ph.D.

Lymphatic massage relieves the pain and swelling in lymph nodes from the build-up of toxins, pollutants, viruses, bacteria and other waste materials.
See ad page 99
28247 Agoura Rd.
Agoura Hills, CA   91301

(818) 707-3126   (818) 707-2787 FAX

MASSAGE THERAPY

Therapeutic massage promotes general well-being and enhances self-esteem. The massage therapist's touch stimulates blood and lymph circulation as well as immune system functioning; reduces muscular tension and swelling of ligaments and tendons; and relieves pain in muscles and joints. Therapists draw on Eastern and/or Western techniques.

John Benedict, N.M.T.

Neuro muscular re-education. Myofascial release. Relief of chronic soft tissue pain and dysfunction. Sports injuries and maintenance.
Topanga   **(310) 712-1219**

Elyse Briggs

Licensed Massage Therapist
Specializing in Prenatal, Thai, Swedish, Deep Tissue and Profound Relaxation.
See ad page 104
ak413@latn.org
BRIGGSBODYWORKS@www.geocities.com/HOTSPRINGS/SPA/8162/
Glendale   **(818) 241-1781**

Ann Marie Gallagher

Hands On: Massage Therapy. Special Kneads. Swedish. Shiatsu. On-Site-Office-Chair-Massage. Stress Management.
4730 Oakwood Ave.
La Canada, CA   91011   **(818) 790-7883**

Golden Touch Massage

Sheri Goldberg
Eclectic, experienced professional practitioner offering Swedish, Myofacial (works tension and chronic spasm out of deep muscle layers), pregnancy massage (relieves lower back pain, swelling & leg pain), Reflexology (vitalizes precise pressure points) and Reiki (facilitates healing & heightens energy flow). A safe, soothing environment that nourishes transformation.

Gift certificates and package discounts available. Out calls to home or office.
3868 Centinela,
Mar Vista/Marina Del Rey, CA   90066
     (310) 397-0977 (310) 479-7792 FAX

Michael Goldstein

Licensed Massage Therapist
18 years experience. My expertise is in joining Deep Tissue Muscle Manipulation and Myofascial Release techniques with Acupressure Massage.
West Los Angeles   **(310) 737-1998**

Martha Hall

Health - Energy - Calm. Prenatal, Swedish and Deep Muscle Massage with Spirit.
West Los Angeles/Santa Monica border
                              (310) 578-5577

Healing Spirit

Lynette Luis & Claudia Auffenberg
Massage Therapy & Bodywork: Let us reduce stress in your work place! Our services will leave you relaxed and rejuvenated. We make office visits & movie set outcalls! See ad page 100
Los Angeles & S. F. Valley
                              (818) 761-4367

Healing Hands, Zsuzsanna Krausz

Now is the time to get your body healthy. Therapeutic massage, deep tissue release and acupressure. Stimulates blood circulation and cleanses by pushing along lymphatic fluids. Give your body a chance to balance with Reiki. Teaching Reiki level I and II. See ad page 118
Redondo Beach   *(310) 373-9682*

Institute for Health

Teresa Rispoli, L.Ac, Ph.D.
Through the healing art of massage variations, tension and pain melt away, anxiety lessens and a heightened sense of well-being overcomes you. See ad page 99
28247 Agoura Rd.
Agoura Hills, CA 91301
     (818) 707-3126   (818) 707-2787 FAX

Penny Layne

Transformational Healing Body Work including therapeutic massage, body wraps, facials, kineseology, Sunrider products, Reiki, crystals and hypnosis. See ad page 109
Los Angeles   *(213) 664-7788*

Amy Kasten, Ms.T.

Massage therapy, reflexology, therapeutic stretching, and home-grown herbs.
Santa Monica mountains
          (310) 455-9971

Kara Masters, M.A.

In Touch: a practice of deepening connection with self and surroundings through massage and movement therapy that center, soothe and invigorate.
See ad page 82
Westside   *(310) 359-5599*

Malibu Massage Center

Massage, therapeutic spa treatments, chiropractic, acupuncture, reflexology, nutritional counseling and energy healing.
21241 Pacific Coast Highway
Malibu, CA 90265
          (310) 456-1953

Diane Miller, Ms.T.

"We are simply a moment of breath."
I offer a uniquely soothing, balancing massage experience combining a variety of techniques, as well as hands-on healing, in the comfort of your own home.
Malibu & Westside   *(310) 456-3041*

Caitlin Philips, Ms.T., CD

Offers a wide variety of body/mind techniques from Eastern to Western, including pre-natal & childbirth assistance. Office located at West Los Angeles/Santa Monica border
          (310) 239-4023

Aryeh Shell

Swedish, Deep-Tissue, Thai and pregnancy massage; through awareness, inquiry, and integration of body, mind and emotions. See ad page 125
Santa Monica   *(310) 939-3408*

Rochelle L. Tepper

Intuitive, deep tissue massage, using structural integration to balance the body/mind. See ad page 101
          (310) 252-0870

Touch Therapy Massage

Touch Therapy Massage offers treatment given by the graduates of The Touch Therapy Institute. We offer a full range of services from Basic Swedish to Lomilomi to Reflexology and much more. 10:00 a.m. to 8:00 p.m. See ad page 78
15720 Ventura Blvd. Suite 101
Encino, CA 91436
     (818) 788-1816   (818) 788-0875 FAX

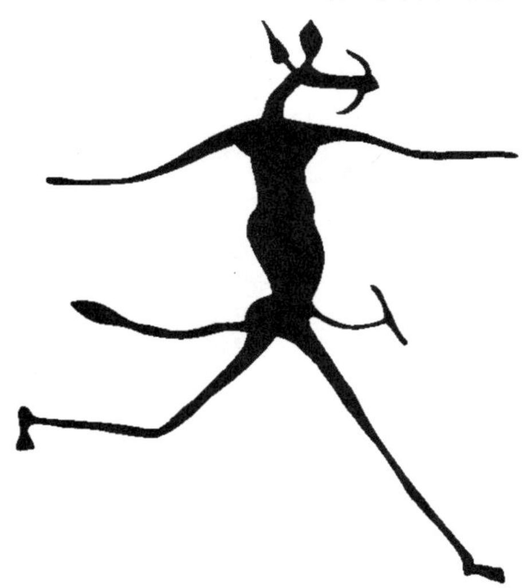

"A little rebellion now and then is a good thing."

—THOMAS JEFFERSON

MEDIATION

*M*ediation is the artful science of bringing differing parties together for constructive resolution. As an alternative to costly litigation, mediation provides a context for voicing legal problems, airing conflicting opinions, and seeking agreeable solutions.

Richard Gottfried M.A., M.F.C.C.

Mediation, Arbitration, Conciliation.

Certified Mediator; shared parenting, divorce, community, commercial.

21070 W. Summit Road
12381 Wilshire Blvd., Suite 200

Topanga	**(310) 455-3804**
West Los Angeles	**(310) 572-4366**

Richard Millen, Attorney

Mediation, Non-Litigation, Conflict Resolution & Legal Consulting

15235 Valley Vista Blvd.
Sherman Oaks, CA   91403

(818) 501-2787

Dena Saxer, M.A., Mediator

Dispute Specialties: neighbor/neighbor, tenant/landlord, consumer/merchant, family inheritance, business partnership.

(310) 455-1936

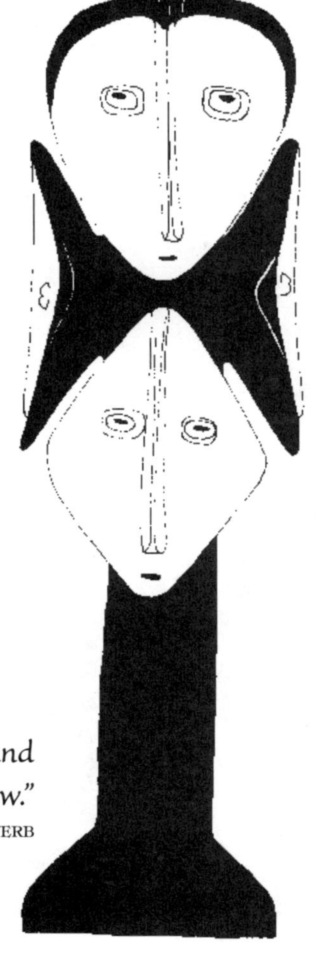

"Stop thinking and talking about it and there is nothing you will not be able to know."
—ZEN PROVERB

MEDITATION STRESS REDUCTION

Meditation practices encourage mental concentration while holding a point of focus. Meditation brings the body, mind and spirit together in the present moment. In this state of mindful awareness, people relax, heal and experience empowerment, balance and feel more centered. The ultimate purpose of this practice is Self knowledge and enlightenment.

Gloria Kamler, M.A.

A Taste of Mindfulness. Stress reduction/relaxation/Jon Kabat-Zinn modeled program. Proven to reduce stress, pain, anxiety, depression. It works! Santa Monica School of Integrated Studies.
See ad page 85
Santa Monica   *(310) 450-4541*

Ordinary Dharma Center

Classes, retreats and workshops in the tradition of Thich Nhat Hanh. Mindfulness and meditation. Buddhist studies. Aikido and non-violence training. Deep ecology process work. See ad page 75
Santa Monica & Warner Springs
(310) 394-6653

Dena Saxer, M.A.

Senior Healing TAO Instructor

Basic Meditation, Sexual Energy Meditation, Iron Shirt Chi Kung, Tai Chi.
(310) 455-1936

Jason Siff

The Skillful Meditation Project
Vipassana Meditation instruction, sitting groups, retreats.
Topanga, Los Angeles & Idyllwild
(323) 223-2470   *(909)659-2649*

Topanga Zen Group

In lineage of Shunryu Suzuki. Sunday morning meditation from 9:00 to 10:30 led by Peter Levitt. Everyone Welcome!
Levgran@aol.com
Topanga   *(310) 455-9404*

The Santa Monica Zen Center

Meditation. See ad page 103
1001 A Colorado Ave.
Santa Monica, CA   90401
(310) 572-9070

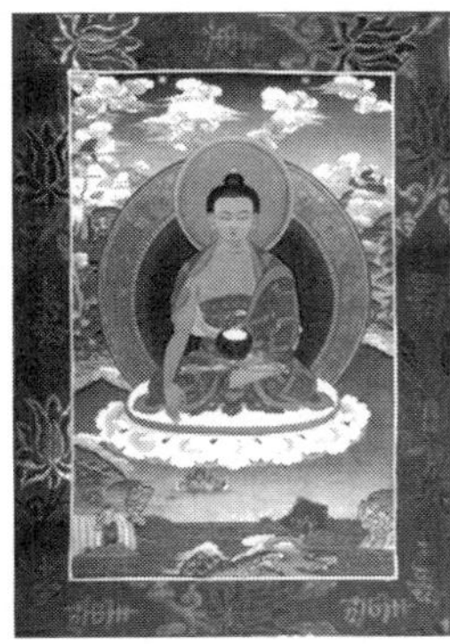

"Without inner peace, it's impossible to have world peace."
—14TH DALI LAMA

MOVEMENT RE-EDUCATION

Ease comes from the Latin 'elbows akimbo.' Disease then literally means not enough elbow room. Movement re-education exercises offer us a direct and primary experience of creating space and ease not only for our elbows but for our bodies, minds and spirits.

ALEXANDER TECHNIQUE

The Alexander Technique, a profound psycho-physical re-education, creates lasting improvement in posture and ease of movement. It has been shown to alleviate persistent back pain, improve breathing and release anxiety stress. Practitioners offer this technique to their clients in a series of lessons.

Charlotte Holtzermann
MFA, NASTAT, CMT

Charlotte offers individual sessions and group classes in Alexander technique, Hatha yoga, Massage and Watsu.
Westside & Topanga
(310) 348-9118 or (310) 455-1000

Lana Spraker, **M.A., NASTAT**
Certified Teacher

Neuro-muscular re-education for peak performance in your daily activities.
See ad page 93
West L.A. & Santa Monica (310) 479-3646

Judith Stransky

Total lasting well-being achieved through renowned mind-body approach: easily improves posture, body habits, alleviates pain. See ad page 105
Santa Monica   (310) 828-5528

FELDENKRAIS®

Feldenkrais method is an innovative movement education system developed by physicist, judo expert and engineer, Dr. Moshe Feldenkrais. It is a highly effective way to acquire and increase movement skills and flexibility as well as potency in self expression and creativity.

Laura McMurray
Certified Feldenkrais Practitioner

Private Lessons & Public Classes. House Calls Welcome.
P.O. Box 481204, L. A., CA   90029
(323) 661-9060

Judith Stransky

Freedom of body - with profound psychophysical benefits - through pleasurable, unique exercises. No practice, all ages. See ad page 105
Santa Monica   (310) 828-5528

PILATES

The Pilates method was developed by German-born Joseph H. Pilates, who was a gymnast, osteopath and boxer. He coupled Eastern (yoga) disciplines with Western strength training to form an exercise system focused on precision, breath and fluid movement.   *Continued*

Kathleen Carman
Certified Pilates Teacher
Mind and Body in Balance. Kathleen specializes in using the Pilates method for rehabilitation as well as re-sculpting the body through specific exercise that strengthen, tone and firm the muscles, increase flexibility, improve over-all posture and structural integrity.
9350 Civic Center Dr., Suite 119
Beverly Hills, CA   90210

(323) 938-6442

Institute for Health
Teresa Rispoli, L.Ac., Ph.D.
Pilates exercise stretches and tones the deep muscles that move the bones and therefore balances and stretches and tones the entire body. Gentle enough for the elderly yet challenging for the athlete.
See ad page 99
28247 Agoura Rd.
Agoura Hills, CA   91301

(818) 707-3126   (818) 707-2787 FAX

Marcia Kellam
Pilates-inspired work-outs in Topanga Canyon. Personalized one-on-one work-out sessions based on the resistance exercise and rehabilitation concepts developed by Joseph Pilates.
See ad page 124
Topanga   (310) 455-0632

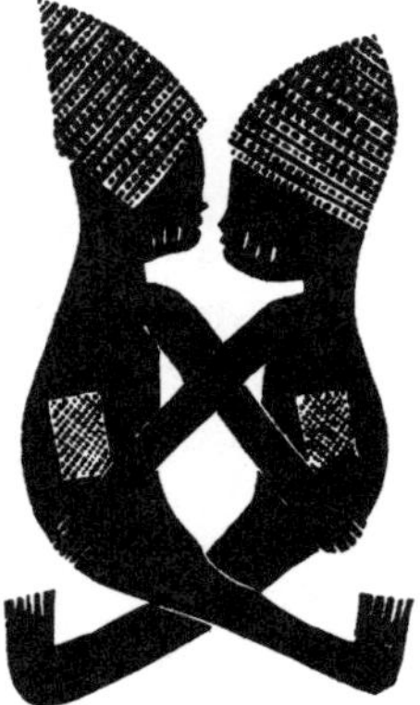

"Lovers don't finally meet somewhere.
They're in each other all along."
—RUMI

NUTRITION
MACROBIOTICS

Nutrition, based in healthy foods, nutritional supplements, and special, fasting and/or cleansing diets, may not be enough. Unless foods and supplements are chemical-free as well as easily metabolized and assimilated, they are of little use to the body. Holistic nutritionists explore with their clients what, how, and where they purchase, store, prepare, consume and feel about foods and supplements. They also consider exercise and self-worth. Nutritionists then act as diagnosticians, guides, teachers, and counselors.

Mindy Boxer, Ph.D., L.Ac., Dipl.Ac., D.Hom.
Nutritional guidance specific to your body
type & constitution. See ad page 109
3301 Ocean Park Blvd.
Santa Monica, CA 90405

(310) 450-9711

Capitol Drugs

A free quarterly newsletter, lecture series &
an educated staff help you make educated
decisions about your healthcare.
See ad page 105
8578 Santa Monica Blvd.
4454 Van Nuys Blvd.

West Hollywood	(310) 289-1125
Sherman Oaks	(818) 905-8338
	(800) 819-9098

Institute for Health

Teresa Rispoli, L.Ac., Ph.D.
Nutritional counseling honors that every
person has different nutritional needs. Let
our trained professionals guide you in
making the right choices for your
individual needs. See ad page 99
28247 Agoura Rd.
Agoura Hills, CA 91301

(818) 707-3126   (818) 707-2787 FAX

Marilyn Joyce, R.D.
Registered Dietician, Author & Speaker
Wholistic Nutrition and Health Educator
& Coach/5 Minutes to Health. A cancer
survivor, world traveler, and master of
yoga, Marilyn discovered that wellness
depends on simplicity and getting back to
basics on every level. She compassionately
inspires clients to positively adopt healthier
diets and lifestyles, employing a wholistic
mind/body/spirit approach.
See ad page 114
West Los Angeles, Nationally & Globally

(310) 391-3130

Cecile Tovah Levin

Los Angeles East West Center for
Macrobiotic Studies: cooking courses,
seminars, workshops and study courses.
See ad page 84

Los Angeles   (310) 398-2228

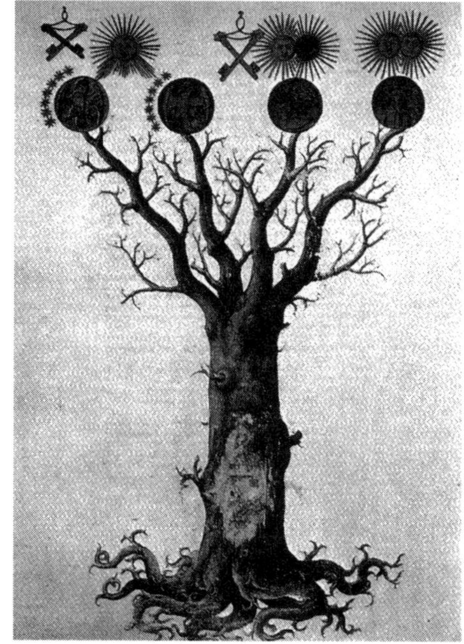

*"Believe nothing, no matter where you read it,
or who said it, no matter if I have said it,
unless it agrees with your own reason and
your own common sense."*
—BUDDHA

PHYSICAL FITNESS

*S*pecific components of fitness include: aerobic (cardiopulmonary) capacity, muscular strength and endurance, flexibility and body composition (proportion of lean vs. fat tissue). Fitness is but one aspect of a complete and balanced wellness program in which an individual consciously moves towards a state of optimal physical, psychological and spiritual health.

Mary Bloom

Home or studio instruction. Women in Transition (35-55), Mature Adults (55+), Stress & Weight Management, and Body Sculpting & Strengthening. See ad page 111

Topanga   **(310) 455-3326**

PHYSICAL THERAPY PAIN MANAGEMENT

Practitioners may use acupuncture, meditation, biofeedback, hypnotherapy, specific diets, exercise and stress reduction techniques to help reduce pain and restore physical health.

Polly Badt

Body Rehab Center for Physical Therapy

The Center provides physical therapy for a variety of disorders, specializing in Orthopedics, Neuromuscular Rehab., Sports Injuries, Manual Therapy and Women's Health. Our goal is for one to function at one's full potential with therapy given on a one on one basis, looking at the individual in a holistic manner.

22601 Pacific Coast Highway
Suite 250, Malibu, CA

(310) 456-8301

SKIN, HAIR & BODY CARE AROMATHERAPY

*T*he practices of facials, make-up artistry, hair-styling, skin and body care enhance a sense of well-being as well as beauty; they incorporate the use of natural products. Aromatherapy also supports a sense of well-being through the therapeutic use of essential fragrant oils, which can be inhaled and/or absorbed through the skin by massage or adding them to water. As oils affect all of the body systems, the results of their use can be felt on physical, emotional and spiritual levels.

The Bey's Garden

A magical world of essential oils, an environment which celebrates the power and beauty of nature's fragrances, a haven of tranquility where people can relax and indulge their senses. See ad page 90

Santa Monica	**(310) 399-5420**
Beverly Hills	**(310) 273-BEYS**

Canyon Hair Studio

Canyon Hair Studio and Skin Care offers clients a charming alternative to a city salon. More like a cozy living room with spectacular state park views, it offers first class services by husband and wife team, Dennis and Sally. See ad page 80

395 South Topanga Canyon Blvd. #204
Topanga, CA   90290

(310) 455-3196

Anna Cirronis
Certified Aromatherapist

"ERBAVIVA": Essential oils are concentrated essences of flowers, fruits, herbs and plants. Using the power of these ancient medicines of the earth, ERBAVIVA creates the purest handcrafted skin care products and soaps.

Topanga   **(310) 455-1984**

Jeneal International Skin Correction & Health Centers

Holistic approach to skin correction and hair regrowth. 25 years dedication to the correction of cosmetic disorders.
See ad page 122

2116 Wilshire Blvd., Suite 103
Santa Monica, CA   90403

(310) 470-0204

Lindy's Facials

Balance body, mind & spirit. Understand how diet, stress & allergies affect the skin. Eliminate blemishes. Reduce wrinkles. See the difference in one visit. Natural products by Lindy. 100% Botanical glygolic peels.

827 Rimpau Blvd.
Los Angeles, CA   90005

(323) 938-6790   (800) 363-HEAL

Sophia Sharpe, Certified
Lymphologist, Reiki Master & Aromatherapist

Discover why the use of the World's Finest Essential Oils support mind, body and emotions through massage, sound, energy and crystal work. See ad page 92

West Los Angeles   **(310) 473-7276**

Tranquility Skin and Body Care
Lori Mass

Create a state of tranquility with our personalized skin and body care treatments and feel yourself transform.

1150 Yale @ Wilshire Blvd., Suite 8
Santa Monica, CA   90403.

(310) 470-0204

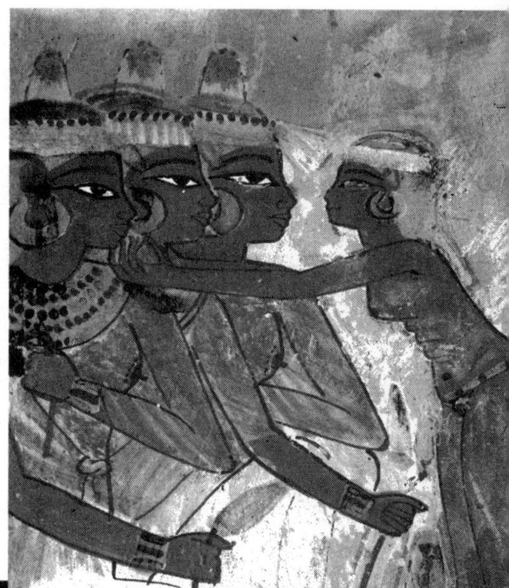

WISDOM TRADITIONS INTERFAITH MINISTRY

Age old traditions inherent in every culture from time immemorial present unique perspectives on the fundamental truths about life: "Who are we?", "Where do we come from?", "What purpose do we have here?" Universal truths are presented; practices for self development and service to Humankind are encouraged.

ASTROLOGICAL ARTS

Astrology, an ancient art and science, maps the interdependence of universal energies between the planets and stars and our own live's forces. Astrology holds to the Hermetic philosopher's adage, "As above, so below," correlating the relationships of energetic, planetary influences with our physical, mental, emotional and spiritual states of consciousness.

Lola Babalon

Experienced psychic, astrologer and tantric shaman offers in-depth counseling, classes and sacred ceremonies. See ad page 116
P.O. Box 645
Topanga, CA   90290

(310) 455-0103

Jean Greer

Astrological Love Connections - a service to locate your soul mates using astrology.
See ad page 114
http://www.jeangreer.com
Greater Los Angeles area   (310) 823-4310

Judith Harte, Ph.D.

Astrological consultant/trained psychotherapist combines mythic astrology with depth psychotherapy. See ad page 109
Westside & Sherman Oaks

(310) 281-7991

COUNCIL

Based on Native American tradition, Council is a way of speaking and listening from the heart. The facilitator develops trust and strengthens communication, decision-making and conflict resolution skills with the individuals in any group. Council aims to bridge differences and foster tolerance among all people.

Catherine Engel

Sisters come, entering our time of menopause, "wise blood." Enter the circle, speaking and listening from the heart, in Council, the ancient way of sacred sharing. See ad page 69
Hollywood & Westside   (310) 459-4528

Michele W. D'Arbanville
Council Facilitator

A method of focus for deeper communication; learn and explore the art of collaborative process. Guidance and mentoring for your family, arts or humanities groups.
By appointment.
Los Angeles   (310) 455-2714

Laurie Schur, L.C.S.W.

Teaching people to draw from their inner wisdom in speaking and listening from the heart.
1315 Westwood Blvd., L.A., CA   90024

(310) 829-5608

Not embracing a particular sectarian dogma, these practitioners provide spiritual counseling from a universal perspective. They practice healing methods grounded in principles at the root of Nature's harmony. Interfaith Ministers are permitted to perform civil services such as baptisms, weddings, and funerals.

Rev. Maya. Brandenberger, Ph.D.
Ordained Unity Minister

Non-denominational worship services, interfaith marriages, ceremonies and rituals. Vision quests. Spiritual Coaching.

Topanga & L.A.   *(310) 455-3129*

Tracy Masington, M.A.
Minister of the Universal Life Church

Personalized wedding ceremonies offering an alternative to dogmatic traditions, designed to reflect the couple's unique spirit.

Throughout the U.S.   *(310) 810-0036*

All indigenous traditions have tribal healers and elders whose consciousness simultaneously spans the three worlds - physical, psychic and spiritual. Shamans use trance techniques, natural substances, dreams and divining methods to uncover truth and perform healings.

Lourdes Chazaro

This is intuitive shamanic work which encourages one's spirit-soul to engage in the process of one's own healing.
See ad page 102

By appointment   *(310) 358-6125*

Lynn Creighton

Lynn Creighton is committed to serving the community through ceremonial experience of awakening to the blessing of life and all the gifts of the great spirit. Purification lodge and vision quests. Solstice/Equinox celebrations.

Northridge   *(818) 886-9006*

G. Lynn Diamond

Celtic Spiritual Shamanic Tradition for personal growth. Individual and group courses.

West Los Angeles   *(310) 391-4088*

Amanda Foulger
Shamanic Services

Counseling, Healing, House Blessings, Talks, Workshops. Los Angeles Area Foundation for Shamanic Studies. Workshop Coordinator and Instructor.

P.O. Box 557, Topanga, CA   90290

(310) 455-3758

Sharon Siegel, Ph.D.

Shamanic, feminine crone work. Pre and post menopausal counseling.
See ad page 116

Los Angeles   *(310) 455-3232*

Healing often is recorded as having taken place in ways such as; the laying of hands, psychic transmissions, psychic surgery and faith healings, which aren't scientific and confound our rational mind. Rather than simply dismissing what the rational mind can't understand, we can choose to open to our creative mind, which feels more comfortable in realms beyond logic. With guidance from our intuition and creative mind, we can investigate different healing approaches.

Judi Castro

Clairvoyant psychic, with help of Angels, transform challenges now, 95% authentic insight, experienced, caring, ethical.

Worldwide   *(818) 344-1429*

Hanna Chusid, Ed.D.

Jewish spiritual practice: women's circles/ life ceremony, mentoring, counseling, dance and meditation. See ad page 111

Westside & San Fernando Valley

(818) 345-3006   *(310) 281-6134*

Nancy Furst

Laying on of Stones. Volunteer Hospice Care. Spiritualist.

(818) 765-5418

Connie Kaplan, M.A.
Universal Life Minister

Using a unique marriage of numerology, astrology, dreams, color therapy, and counseling, I help people remember their Soul's incarnational intent. The result: radical awe of life and deep happiness.
Santa Monica

(310) 451-2157

Jan Kershaw, RM, DHP, HSLHM

Classes on Clairvoyant Development/ Individual Consultations. The Healing Sanctuary: A collective of Healers & Therapists. Inquiries Welcome.
Hollywood

(323) 860-6676

The Labyrinth
Norma Thompson Hollis

Group and individual spiritual teachings.
Inglewood

(310) 671-7136

YOGA

Yoga, meaning balance, is the Eastern spiritual science of self-improvement. Techniques involve bringing one's whole nature into harmony. Practice results in relaxed strength and increased vitality. Various Yoga methods focus through; Mind (Raja), Heart or Devotional (Bakti), Energetic (Kundalini), and Hatha (Breath/Physical postures). Hatha Yoga, in particular, has gained contemporary popularity due to its emphasis on balanced health, breath and relaxation.

Kristi Foster, Yin Yoga

Group or private yoga classes at your home or office, to de-stress your body and mind, while guiding you and your colleagues into finding the courage and strength that lead to enhanced relationships, clarity, efficiency and creativity.
Westside & Downtown   (310) 828-5831

Aryeh Shell

Cultivate your practice through concrete, passionate, immediate felt experience. Ongoing classes and private sessions.
See ad page 125
Santa Monica   (310) 939-3408

Sivananda Yoga Vedanta Center

Yoga and Meditation. First Drop-In Class Free! Daily Drop-In Classes. Beginner's Courses. Yoga Retreats. Teacher's Training Courses. Call for Free Brochure!
LosAngeles@sivananda.org
http://www.sivananda.org/lacenter.htm
1746 Abbott Kinney Blvd.
Venice, CA 90291

(310) 822-9642

Theosophy (Raja Yoga)

The United Lodge Of Theosophists provides a basis for understanding Reincarnation, Karma and Universal Brotherhood. Study of ancient and modern science, philosophy and religion in the light of the original writings of H.P. Blavatsky and William Q. Judge. Call to inquire about free classes (in English and Spanish) and local study groups.
http:www.ULT.org
Theosophy Hall
245 West 33rd St., Los Angeles, CA 90007
(213)748-7244   (213)748-0634 FAX

> *"Never will I seek nor receive private, individual salvation; Never will I enter into final peace alone; but forever, and everywhere, will I live and strive for the redemption of every creature throughout the world."*
>
> *Kwan Yin's Pledge*

Yoga Garden

Ashtanga and Iyengar influenced Hatha Yoga in beautiful garden setting. Small group classes and private instruction. All levels welcome. Yoga to lift your heart, enlighten your mind, and open your body. See ad page 70
Topanga   **(310) 455-7522**

Yoga West

Yogi Bhajan. Director Sat Kirin. Kundalini yoga, healing arts, meditation, internationally certified teachers' trainings, pre natal, weekend retreats and seminars. Call for more information.
1535 S. Robertson Blvd.L.A., CA   90035
(310) 552-4647

Yoga Works

150 classes/week 7 days/week. Beginning through advanced classes. Also specializing in pre-natal, easy does it and seniors.
1426 Montana Ave. 2nd Floor,
Santa Monica, CA 90403
2215 Main St., Santa Monica, CA   90405
(310) 393-5150

The Love Temple

Awaken you to your divinity. Expand your ecstatic energies, open your higher chakras and enter into extended states of bliss. Holistic healing with ancient Indian yogic practices. Transformation through the healing Power of Love. See ad page 116
LuminaLove@aol.comwww.thatmall.com/love
Bel Air   **(310) 393-5150**

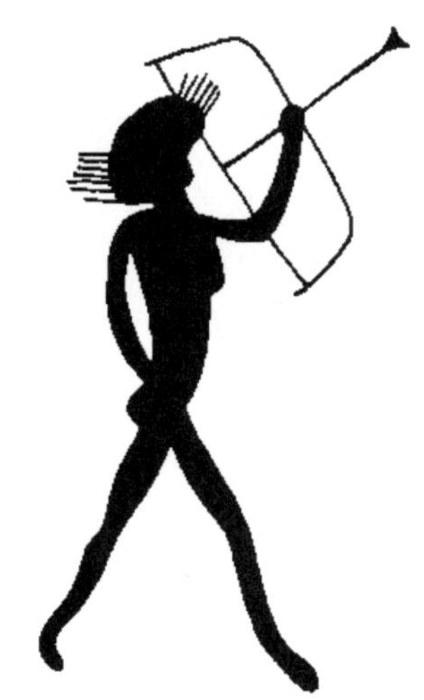

Specialty Providers & Services

Books & Specialties

Bodhi Tree Bookstore, Inc.

One of the world's finest collections of instructive and challenging spiritual books from all disciplines, Eastern and Western. We also have a fine selection of incense, New Age audio/video, greeting cards and gifts. Ask for our Bodhi Tree Book Review Magazine. See ad page 113
bodhitree@bodhitree.com
8585 Melrose Avenue
West Hollywood, CA   90069

(310) 659-1733 or (800) 825-9798

The Old Age Metaphysical Country Store

Crystals and minerals, metaphysical and holistic books, music, incense, essential oils, candles, jewelry, Egyptian art and weekly meditation classes. See ad page 117
www.metaphysical-store.com
7152 Alabama Avenue
Canoga Park, CA   91303

(818) 883-7115

Spiral Staircase Bookstore

A unique esoteric bookstore with unusual gifts, new age music, candles, oils and incense. See ad page 81
128 Old Topanga Canyon Rd.
Topanga, CA   90290

(310) 455-3370

Thunderbolt Books

The new metaphysical book store with unique art, special candles and gifts. See ad page 126
512 Santa Monica
Santa Monica, CA   90401

(310) 899-9279

Assisi

With our present culture's emphasis on the body and its shape, much anxiety and illness has ensued. Assisi clothing designs, non-constricting, free flowing and versatile, free the wearer from those obsessive concerns enabling contact with one's interior rhythm. Hannah Rappaport. See ad page 79
Los Angeles   **(818) 883-4148**

Busy Bee Hardware

Don Kidson. Juice Prophet. Juicers and health books. Water filters, radon testers and amsoil auto products. Raw juice lectures on Tuesdays at 7:00 p.m.
Living Light
Busy Bee Hardware
1457 12th St., Santa Monica, CA   90401
1521 Santa Monica Blvd.
Santa Monica, CA   90404

(310) 395-1158

Cleaner by Nature

The Natural Alternative to Dry Cleaning.
2407 Wilshire Blvd.
11919 Wilshire Blvd.
Santa Monica   **(310) 315-1520**
Brentwood   **(310) 914-4504**

Imagine the Light

Genvieve Laycock Wallis, Celebration Consultant
Engage your own imagination in creating parties, events and celebrations.
geni@artnet.net

(310) 827-7854

Emperors College and Daniel Freeman Marina Hospital Acupuncture Program

Comprehensive medical care, Acupuncture and complementary therapies for inpatients.

(800) 356-2824

Guild of Healers

Seminars held for Service organizations and corporations for the purpose of self-healing and empowerment through Holistic Health Care techniques.

(310) 459-3044

Highland Hall Waldorf School

"Education as an Art" Toddler playgroups, Pre-K, Kindergarten, Grades 1 - 12. Barbara Eriksen, Director of Enrollment.

17100 Superior St., Northridge, CA 91325

(818) 349-1394

Home Away Home

Quality Waldorf style childcare. Ages 4-9. "It is clear to us that Luca is completely understood... in a way that he wouldn't be anywhere else."

Topanga, CA

(310) 455-7026

IPSB: Institute for Psycho-Structural Balancing

A school of holistic body therapy. Also offering IPSB's new Oriental Body therapy programs: Qi Gong and Acupressure. 150 hour program, 500 hour program. Professional Certification.

See ads pages 71 & 87

3767 Overland Blvd., Suite 103
Los Angeles, CA

(310) 815-3675

Cecile Tovah Levin

Los Angeles East West Center for Macrobiotic Studies: cooking courses, seminars, workshops and study courses. See ad page 84

Los Angeles

(310) 398-2228

Seven Arrows

Seven Arrows is a non-profit educational center dedicated to enriching your child's creative mind. See ad page 110

15601 Sunset Blvd.
Pacific Palisades, CA 90272

(310) 454-7277

The Touch Therapy Institute

The Touch Therapy Institute gives the student an opportunity to learn a profession where he or she may use body, mind and spirit to facilitate health, well-being and a better quality of life for self and client and, at the same time, earn a good living. We offer training for beginners as well as continuing education of professionals currently practicing in the field. See ad page 120
www.wholistictouch.com

15720 Ventura Blvd. Ste. 101
Encino, CA   91436

(818) 788-0824   (818) 788-0875 FAX

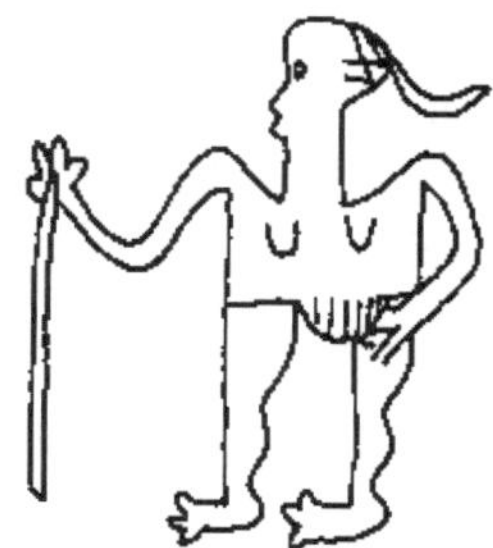

"The most beautiful thing we can experience is the mysterious. It is the source of all true art and science."

—ALBERT EINSTEIN

All Pro Health Foods

A family owned and operated business for over 40 years. At All Pro, we are dedicated to customer service and qualified nutritional guidance. Our goal is the commitment to self-improvement, wellness and a high quality of life.
847 Via De La Paz Pacific Palisades, CA 90272
(310) 454-7457

Co-Opportunity

Santa Monica's Homegrown Natural Food Grocer...we are a full service natural food store specializing in Gourmet/Organic Produce, Vitamins & Supplements, Natural Body Care Products, Macrobiotics, Bulk Foods & Herbs. We also feature a full service Deli soon expanding to include Juice & Coffee Bars and fresh fruit smoothies.
1525 Broadway, Santa Monica, CA 90404
(310) 451-8902

Country Natural Food Store

Be healthy and go country natural.
See ad page 106
415 South Topanga Canyon Blvd.
Topanga, CA 90290
(310) 455-3434

Follow Your Heart

The complete natural foods market, vitamin and body care store. Feel at home dining in our natural food cafe.
21825 Sherman Way, Canoga Park, CA
(818) 348-3240

Gourmet Alchemy

Organic whole foods for all types and tastes. Full service food and home consultations. Special needs for all food concerns.
See ad page 110
Los Angeles & Malibu   **(310) 457-7124**

Grassroots

Fresh organic produce and groceries. Homeopathics, herbs, vitamins, cosmetics, books and free seminars. Natural market and kitchen since 1968. See ad page 86
1119 Fair Oaks Ave., So. Pasadena, CA 91030
(626) 799-0156

Kowalke Family Sprouts

Family sprouts organically grown. Grown to be the best. See ad page 83
Topanga   **(310) 455-1901**

Pacific Coast Greens

Full service deli, bakery, organic produce, hormone & antibiotic free meat, farm-raised fish, organic coffee & juice bar, vitamins, cruelty-free cosmetics, catering & delivery. Senior Discounts. Open 7 days a week from 9 a.m. to 9 p.m. See ad page 82
22601 Pacific Coast Highway Malibu, CA 90265
(310) 456-0353 (310) 456-8606 FAX

Topanga Quality Honey

Honey. Royal jelly honey. Royal jelly. Pollen. Beeswax. BBQ sauce. Available at Bennett S. Honey Farm and Pacific Coast Greens. See ad page 111
P.O. Box 175, Piru, CA 93040
(800) 521-2889

The Vitamin Barn

Something Healthy Inside. All Natural Brands. Discount Prices. See ad page 94
23823 West Malibu Rd., Malibu, CA 90265
(310) 317-4833

Whole Foods Market

A supermarket with a whole new perspective. See back page for our nearest locations...
(888) SHOP-WFM

Yoganics

Yoganics offers weekly home delivery of organic fruits and vegetables designed to suit your household and budget. We also offer organic groceries including grains, pastas, oils, honey, nuts and much more!
See ad page 89
Los Angeles County   **(213) 617-3888**
Orange County   **(888) 4YOGANICS**

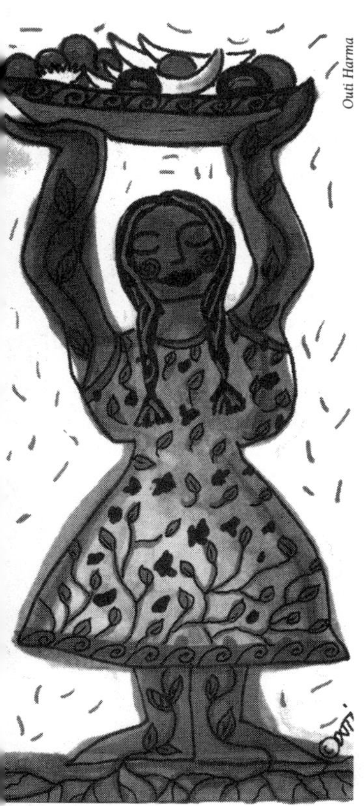

uisine is when things taste like hemselves. —CURNOSKY

Comfort Cafe

Located at Fred Segal. Food for your Life.
See ad page 75
420 Broadway, Santa Monica, CA 90401

(310) 395-6252

Beverly Hills Juice

Over 20 years creating fresh, organic, cold press juices. Special delicious synergistic blends promote health and vigor. Wholesale and retail.
8382 Beverly Blvd.
West Hollywood., CA 90048   (323) 655-8300

Froggy's Topanga Fish Market & Restaurant

Fresh fish and wholesome atmosphere. Open 7 days a week. 5:00 p.m. to 9:30 p.m. Sunday through Thursday and 5:00 p.m. to 10:00 p.m. Friday and Saturday. See ad page 77
1105 North Topanga Canyon Blvd.
Topanga, CA   90290

(310) 455-1728

Inn of the 7th Ray

A restaurant designed around an old Topanga church. Creekside dining under sycamores. Natural food cuisine. See ad page 81
128 Old Topanga Canyon Rd.
Topanga, CA   90290

(310) 455-1311

Jamba Juice

Smoothies & Juices & Healthy Snacks.
See ad page 89
21915 Ventura Blvd.
Woodland Hills, CA   91364

(818) 888-2582

Love and Serve

Vegetarian restaurant. Mock tuna, barbecued tofu, neatloaf and un-chicken. See ad page 100
1110 Gayley Ave.
Westwood, CA

(310) 209-1055

Nawab of India

House of Exotic Indian Food. Saturday and Sunday all you can eat champagne lunch buffet. Food to go. Delivery. Catering.
See ad page 94
1621 Wilshire Blvd.
Santa Monica, CA   90403

(310) 829-1106

Nyala Ethiopian Cuisine

Ethiopian cuisine originating from East Africa. A Unique culinary experience. Exotic spices marinated into lamb, beef and chicken. Specializing in vegetarian. See ad page 98
1076 South Fairfax Ave.
Los Angeles, CA.

(323) 936-5918

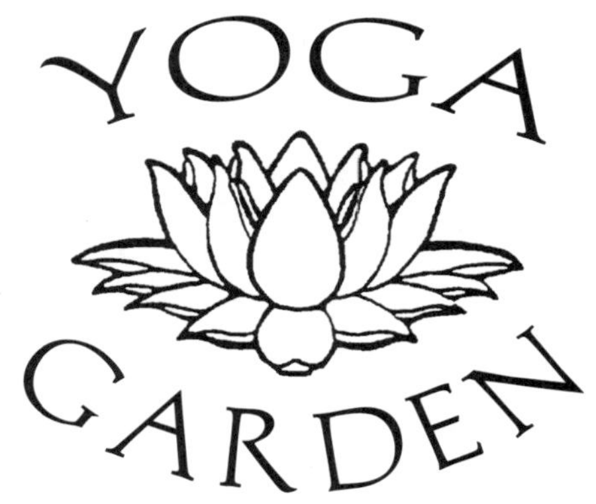

YOGA GARDEN

MARY-BETH DEMERS
Certified Yoga Instructor

All levels of Hatha Yoga Instruction including

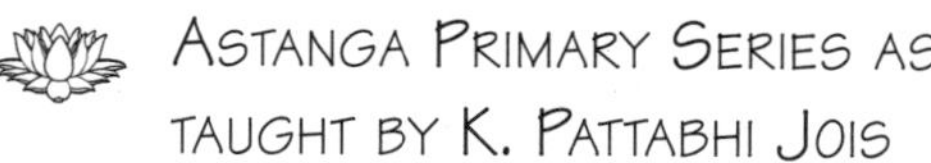 Astanga Primary Series as taught by K. Pattabhi Jois

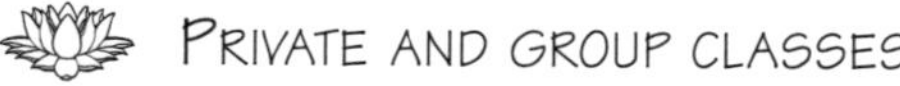 Private and group classes

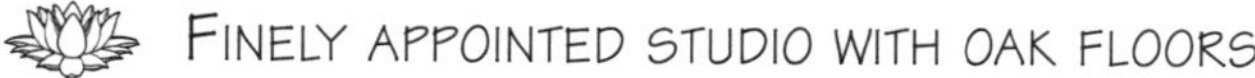 Finely appointed studio with oak floors

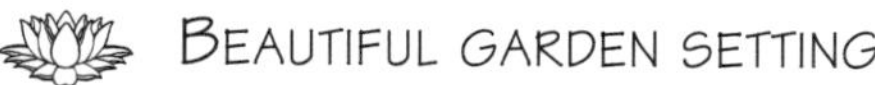 Beautiful garden setting

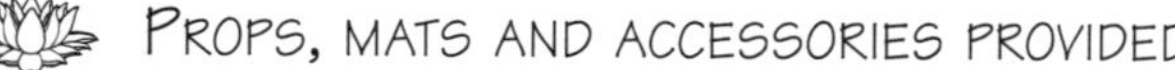 Props, mats and accessories provided

HOURS: BY APPOINTMENT/GROUP CLASSES TO BE ANNOUNCED

1418 Bonnell Drive · Topanga, CA   310·455·7522

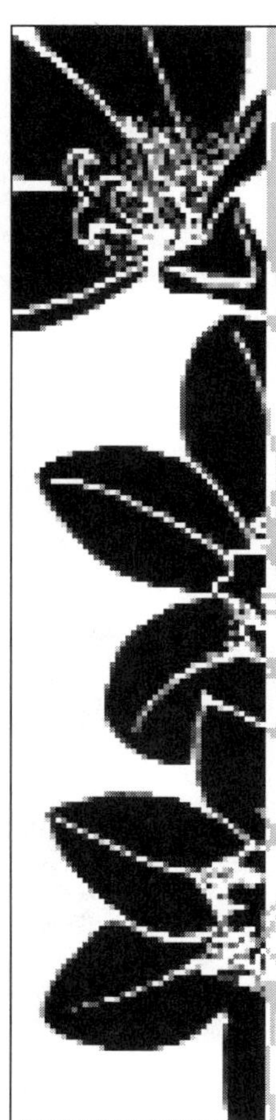

Are You Looking For A Holistic Physician?

Shera Raisen, M.D. is Board Certified in Family Practice and offers both western traditional medicine and alternative therapies. Dr. Raisen combines old-fashioned bedside manner with modern laboratory testing.

§ Care For The Whole Family
§ Women's Health Care & Gynecology, Including Menopause and Natural Hormones
§ Preventative Health Care
§ Nutritional Therapies, Herbs and Functional Medicine Testing

Call for Appointment

Dr. Shera Raisen
900 Wilshire Blvd., Suite 450
Santa Monica, CA 90401

310 394 7277

MA MFCC LICENSE NO. 8698

mind
maryana palmer
body

PSYCHOTHERAPY

Spirit

Individual, couples, family and group therapy specializing in life threatening illness, visualization and guided imagery and bereavement

Telephone 310.455.1743
Offices in Encino & West L.A.

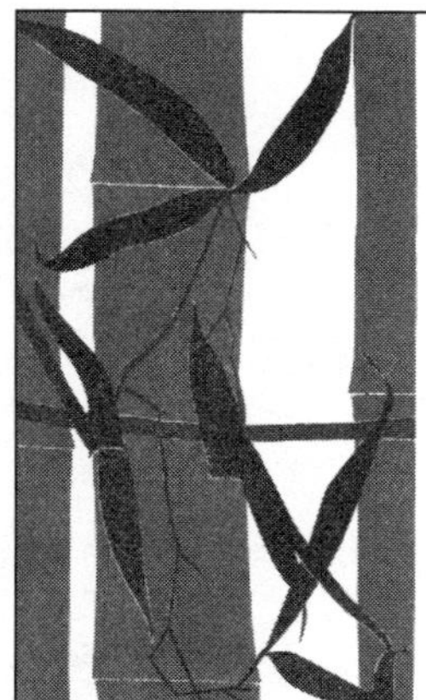

FORRESTPAINTER *design*

**INTERIOR AND LANDSCAPE DESIGN
PSYCHOLOGICAL
AND HUMAN FACTORS**

Constance Forrest, Psy.D.
226 Sherman Canal Venice California 90291
310 822 3640 telephone and facsimile

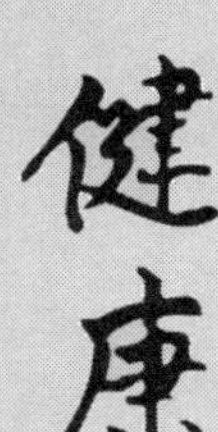

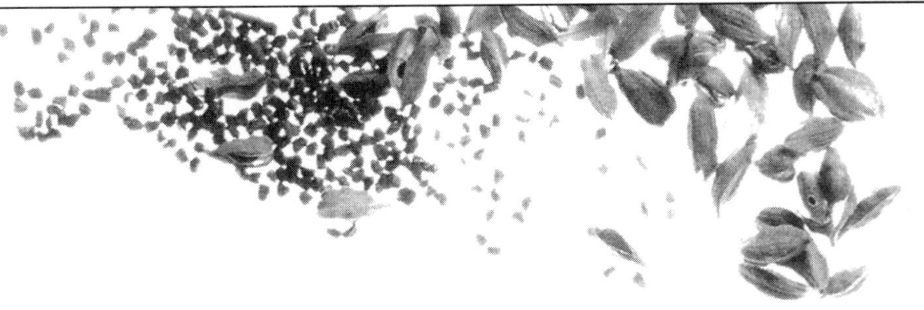

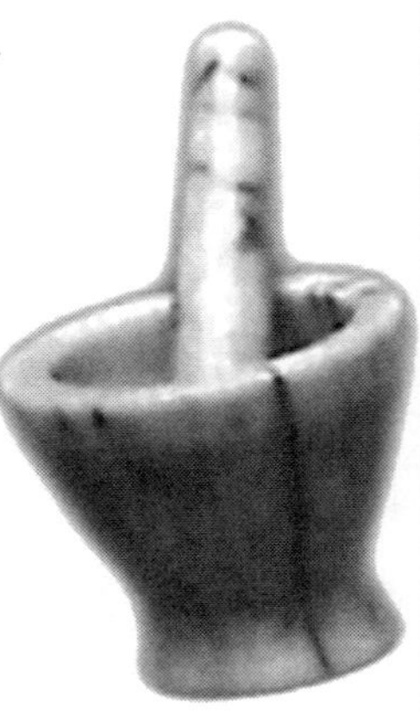

PEACE OF MIND

You buy insurance to secure your loved ones and to gain peace of mind for yourself.
How can you be sure you're getting the best value for your insurance dollar?
The sad truth is most people pay too much for too little when it comes to insurance.
As a broker, I work for you, not the insurance companies. In a matter of minutes
I can show you how to lower your premiums and increase your benefits.
Don't overpay. Call for a no obligation quote and free portfolio analysis.

HEALTH INSURANCE
LIFE INSURANCE
LONG TERM CARE INSURANCE
DISABILITY INSURANCE
ANNUITIES
CA LICENSE #0B49283

JOHN FAZAKERLEY
ESTATE SPECIALIST
(310) 854-0379

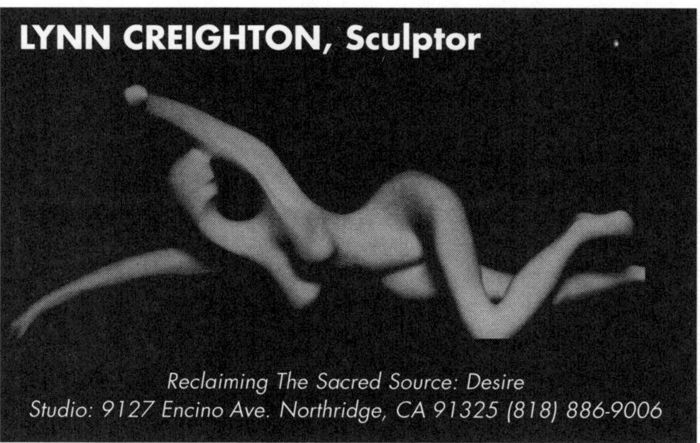

LYNN CREIGHTON, Sculptor

Reclaiming The Sacred Source: Desire
Studio: 9127 Encino Ave. Northridge, CA 91325 (818) 886-9006

LAUREN S. FEDER, M.D.

GENERAL PRACTICE IN HOMEOPATHIC MEDICINE

CHILDREN, ADULTS, PREGNANCY

Dr. Feder has lectured extensively on homeopathy and has been featured in magazines, the internet (parenthoodweb.com), and on television. In addition to hosting her own series of workshops, she is involved in holistic health, natural parenting, and breastfeeding issues. Dr. Feder has a private practice in Beverly Hills, California. Look for her **XCM** line of homeopathic products coming soon!

415 N. Crescent Dr., Suite 100
Beverly Hills, CA 90210

By Appointment (310) 247-1531

Sacred Power Movement

Martial Arts, Energy Cultivation and healing

with

Mathew Cohen

Seminars, private and classes available

310-392-6788

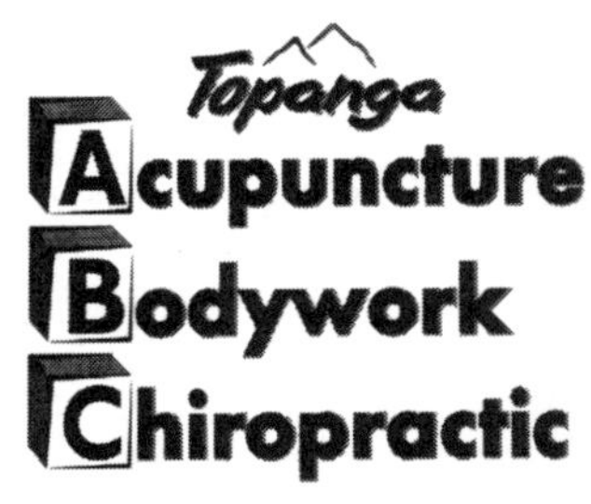

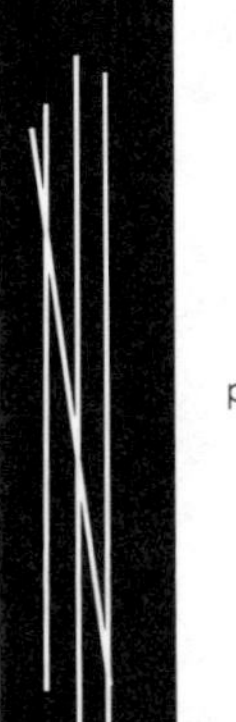

Kartar Diamond
Certified Feng Shui Consultant

FENG SHUI SOLUTIONS: ANCIENT WISDOM
FOR BETTER MODERN LIVING

Improve your home and work environment with ancient energetic principles of design and placement. Your physical surroundings impact your health, success, and relationships. Have a traditionally-trained specialist help you harness the opportunities and balance that you deserve. Long-distance internet clients welcome.

http://www.loop.com/~kartar

Southern California   (310) 820-7891

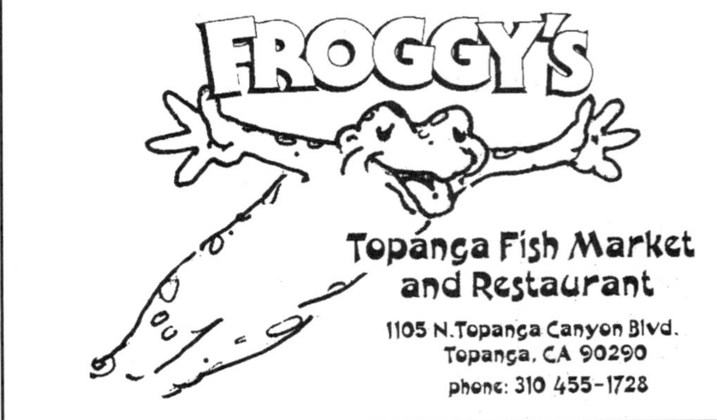

In Touch

Massage and Movement Therapy
Kara Masters, MA • 310 359 5599

Rosanne Mangio
Certified
310 • 459 • 3044

- Vibrational Healing Massage Therapy
- Footbone Massage
- Reiki
- Acupressure
- Essential Oil Therapy
- Fluid Body Coaching
- Abdominal Massage
- Animal Treatments

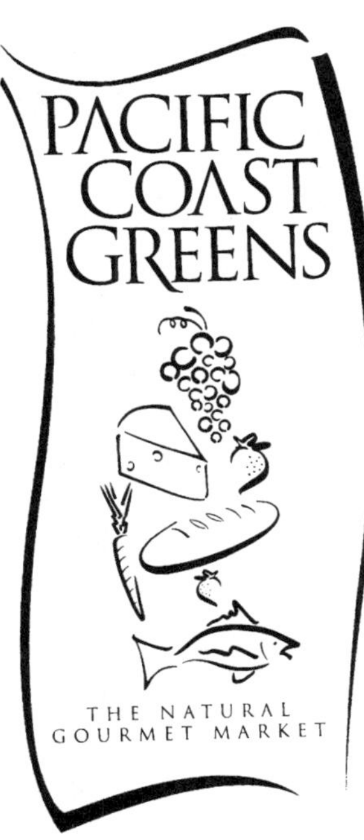

FULL SERVICE DELI

BAKERY

ORGANIC PRODUCE

HORMONE & ANTIBIOTIC-FREE MEAT

FARM RAISED FISH

ORGANIC COFFEE & JUICE BAR

VITAMINS

CRUELTY FREE COSMETICS

CATERING

DELIVERY

22601 PACIFIC COAST HIGHWAY
MALIBU. CA 90265
PHONE (310) 456-0353, FAX (310) 456-8606
OPEN 7 DAYS A WEEK, 9 A..M.-9 P.M.

Ayn Cates

Aura Soma Practitioner

Auro-Soma's colour oils glimmer like jewels in the sunshine. They are actually tools designed to gradually unlock your greatest gifts. Over the past eight years, Ayn Cates has often heard clients remark that after having a session they feel comfortable in their body for the first time. Others achieve emotional equilibrium after years of unhappiness. Many people become aware of their life path. Some individuals, through the use of colour, are able to contact their higher Selves.

For private appointments contact
310-289-7872 Beverly Hills
For courses or more information contact
Ayn Cates, Ph.D. 310-578-5507

Kowalke Family Sprouts

Organically Grown
Grown to be the Best

Nurit Berger

1956 Old Topanga Canyon Road
310-455-1901   310-455-3121 fax
email-kowalke@earthlink.net

e·l·i·x·r

Tonics & Teas

8612 Melrose Ave. Los Angeles, CA 90069

310-657-9300

www.elixrnet.com

Los Angeles WORKSHOP(S) WITH
SOUND, COLOR & CRYSTALS

Exploring the language of the Soul

Presented By: Fred Thompson - Int'l Teacher of Sound, Color & Essence

---

Deepening Clairvoyant Perception Using Color & Sound

Fred with Jan Kershaw - Renowned Clairvoyant Teacher & Healer from Scotland
Eve. Intro.: June 17 or July 2, 1998 / Workshop(s) - June 20-21 or July 4-5, 1998

Tuning In with Sound & Color to promote Self-Healing

Fred with Amy Thakurdas - Professional Musician & Sound Healing Practitioner
Workshop(s) - August 1 - 2 or November 7 -8 , 1998

Energy Intensive with Color, Sound & Silence

described as "Climbing the Mountain without Leaving the Room"
Fred with Hernan Quinones - Spiritual Teacher & Healer from Peru
Workshop - August 29 - 30, 1998

Soul, Sound & Rhythm   (Feb. 13-14, 1999)

Fred & Glen Velez - Recording Artist & World's Foremost Hand Drummer

Soul, Sound & Rhythm - European Tour of Ancient Energy Sites

(May 17 - June 7, 1999) -   Fred & Glen Velez

For more information call: Fred (310) 306-6265
P.O. Box 88039, L.A., CA 90009

AURA-SOMA COLOR THERAPEUTICS
A Unique Color System

Aura-Soma is living color. Color, supported by the energies of plants & crystals, can restore, revitalize & rebalance ourselves at all levels

YOU ARE THE COLOR YOU CHOOSE

For products and consultations visit Healing Waters at
136 N. Orlando Ave., Los Angeles   (213) 651-4656

For training in this unique Color Therapeutic system
or product via mail order, contact:
Fred Thompson (310) 306-6265, P.O. Box 88039, L.A., CA 90009

Fred Thompson - Director of Aura-Soma, USA
Faculty Member, International Academy of Color Therapeutics at "Dev Aura," UK. Certification Instructor for all courses

INTRO.'S	INTERMEDIATE
Monthly	July 8-12, 1998
	Sept. 18-22, 1998

FOUNDATION	ADVANCED
July 24-28, 1998	Sept. 4-9, 1998
Sept. 11-15, 1998	Nov. 20-24, 1998
Oct. 16-20, 1998	
Jan. 29- Feb. 2, 1999	
April 2-6, 1999	

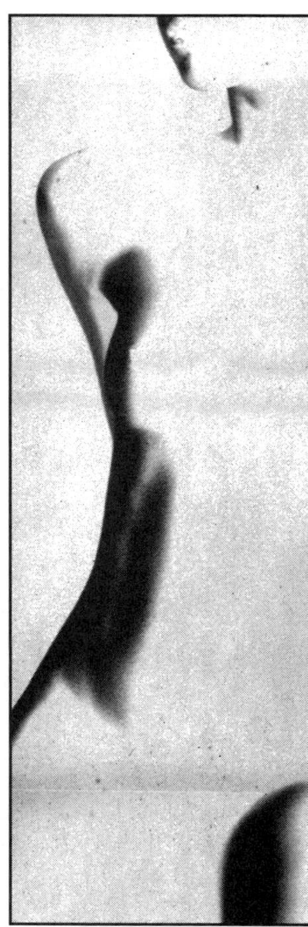

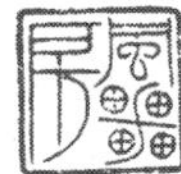

Eileen Hamsa Henry, L.Ac., O.M.D., Ph.D.
Doctor of Oriental Medicine
Diplomatic National Board of Acupuncture
Orthopedics

Acupuncture	*Clinical Nutrition*
Herbology	*Wellness Counseling*

Brentwood Center for Wellness
11611 San Vicente Blvd., Suite 650
Los Angeles, CA 90049
310-826-8606

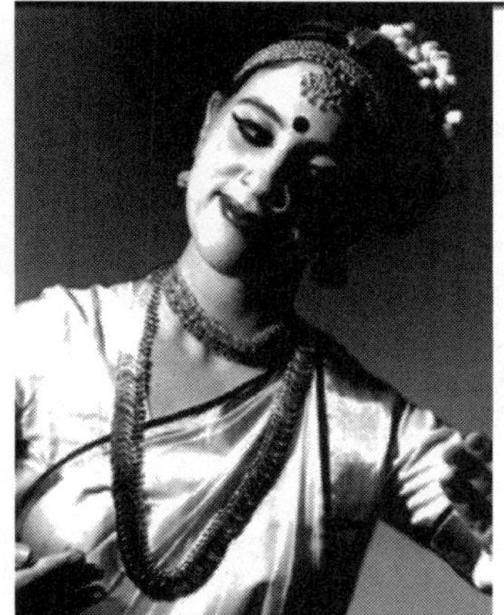

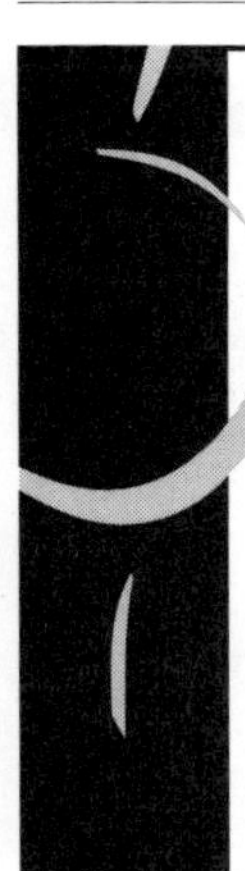

Radiant Health

Michael J. Maguire L.Ac.

Acupuncture
Herbal Medicine
Nutrition

4003 Michael Ave., Los Angeles CA 90066
Los Angeles 310-306-4771/888-220-4153
Malibu 310-457-4714

radhealth@earthlink.net

Tim Ellis Constructions

General contractor committed to not using old growth trees. Specializing in seismic resistant construction and hillside construction. Recycles all usable waste. Utilizing newest technology in wood product engineering to reduce impact on the remaining native environment.

(310) 455-0020
tellis1@earthlink.net

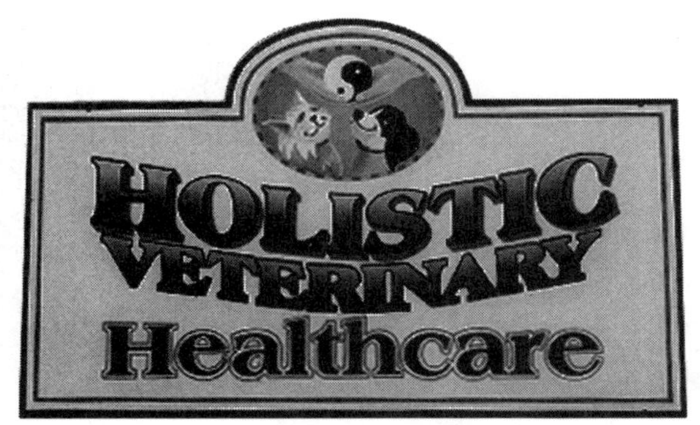

Dr. Marc Bittan, D.V.M.

Acupuncture, Herbs,
Homeopathy, Chiropractic

Special Interest In Geriatrics
Acute & Chronic Disorders Treated

11673 National Boulevard
Los Angeles, California 90064
Tel 310.231.4415
Fax 310. 231.4418
www.netfopets.com

Institute For *Health*

28247 Agoura Road, Agoura Hills, CA 91301

Colon Therapy

Do you suffer from the following:
- *Digestive Disorders, Gas, Bloating*
- *Weight Control & Eating Disorders*
- *Fatigue & Weakness, Headaches*
- *Fasting & Internal Cleansing*

Let us take you to a new level of Health. Feel great! People can eliminate as much as 10 to 40 lbs. over a series of treatments by cleansing the colon. We use purified sterile water and disposable equipment. We also replace a human strain of beneficial bacteria.

Acupuncture

Teresa Rispoli, Ph.D., L.Ac. has practiced Homeopathic and holistic medicine since 1978 and works on boosting the immune system.

Allergies: Homeopathic method of desensitization to food & environmental allergens. Also uses the NAET method.

Allergies	*Arthritis*
Constipation	*Hair Growth*
Diabetes	*Infertility & PMS*
Anxiety	*Stop Smoking*
Drug Abuse	*Asthma*
Pain	*Hypertension*
Impotency	*Hormone Imbalance*

BIO-Evaluation—Homeopathy

Nutrition Guide

Widespread degenerative disease, cancer, cardiovascular disease, arthritis, and other complaints point to a basic gap in public understanding of how to achieve and maintain a state of true health.

Latest supplements: Noni, MSM, Colloidal Minerals, Arise & Shine, Awareness, Chinese Herbs, Calorad, Zinaxin

STATE OF THE ART LAB TESTING
- *Allergy (Food/Environmental) Tests*
- *Liver Detox Capacity Test*
- *Nutrient/Mineral Test*
- *Bacteria, Candida, parasite Test*

Cranio Sacral/Emotional Release, Chiropractic, Lymph Massage, Pilates Based Exercise, Iridology

(818) 707-3126   www.globalhealing.com

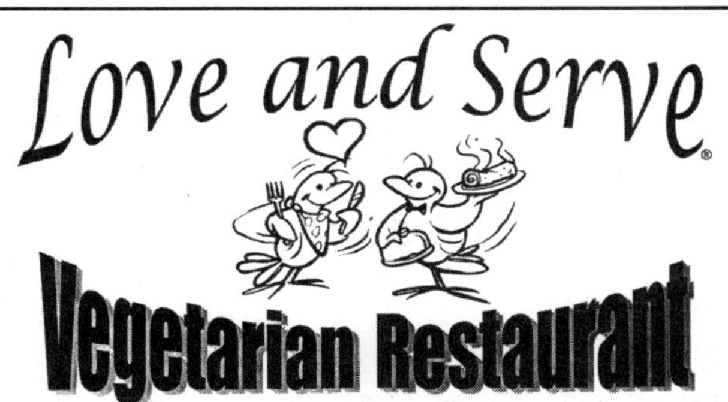

Love and Serve®
Vegetarian Restaurant
1110 Gayley and Wilshire (near 405/UCLA)
310-209-1055

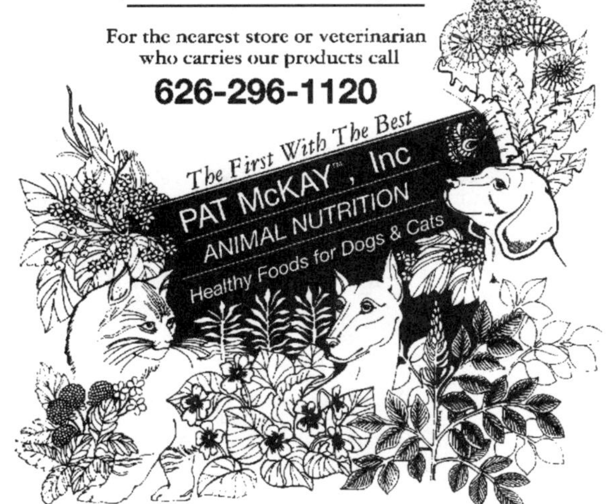

The First With The Best
PAT McKAY™, Inc
ANIMAL NUTRITION
Healthy Foods for Dogs & Cats

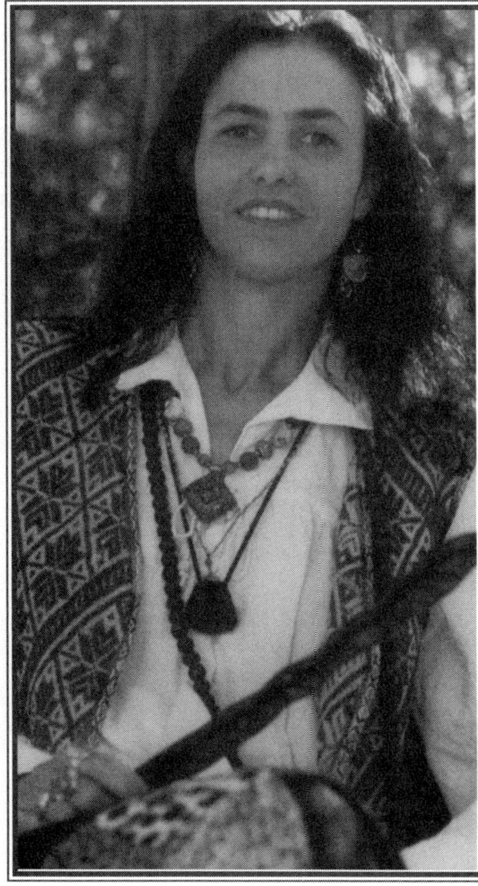

Lourdes Chazaro

COLORPUNCTURE THERAPY
SHAMANIC HEALING

Your real essence is your Soul.
Without Soul a person loses the ability to enjoy life.
Our Inner expression is the Spirit within.
Without Soul and Spirit true happiness cannot be found.
With color and light I heal your Soul and Spirit:
your life can change forever.
Letting go of the past with compassion and forgiveness, we free our
soul like an eagle flying through the rainbow in the sky.

Lourdes Chazaro

BY APPOINTMENT
310-455-1904

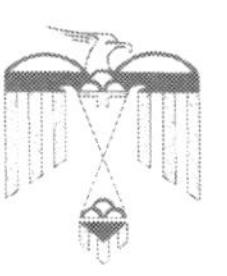

Kerry Hill

Doctor of Chiropractic

Family Chiropractic Care including:

- Non-force treatment for children and pregnancy
- Individual nutritional and lifestyle programs designed for optimum health and vitality — including infant nutrition
- State of the art assessments
- Interest free credit card financing

1411 5th Street

Suite 405

Santa Monica, CA 90401

Telephone 310.458.0400

Santa Monica Zen Center

1001 A Colorado Ave.
Santa Monica, CA 90401

For Further Information of Meditation Times, Instruction and Programs, Call
310-572-9070

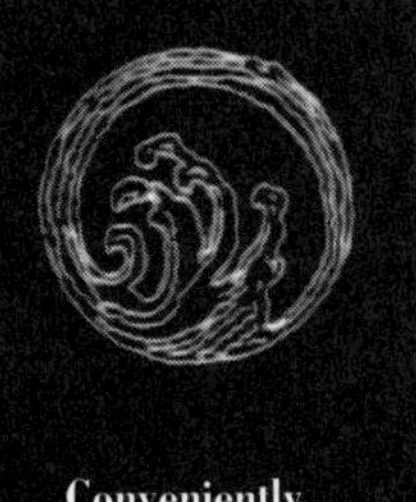

Jeffrey Garson Shapiro, HD PhD

Doctor of Homeopathy
Flower Essence Therapist
Holistic Health and Nutrition

Phone: 310-458-6099
Fax: 310-394-7114

DISCOVER SEVEN ARROWS CULTURAL CENTER
Studio Arts, Music, language, Dance, Science, and Building, Theatre, Athletics, Early Childhood Arts
Creative Classes
in the Woods of Temescal Canyon, Pacific Palisades
Serving Ages 1-Adult
Call Now for a Brochure
310/454-7277
Seven Arrows is a non-profit educational center dedicated to enriching your child's creative mind

Gourmet Alchemy
Babette
Whole Foods—Transformed into elegantly simple meals in your home
Shopping Service, Freezer/Refrigerator Stocking and Equipment Advisement
310–455–3518 Phone 310–457–7124 Fax

Nurturing The Human Spirit in Nature
Counseling that takes place in an Office or out in Nature . Specializing in therapy with Children, Adolescents, Parents and Families. Individually or in groups.
Please call
Patty Factor, MFCC
for more information
(310)588-0786

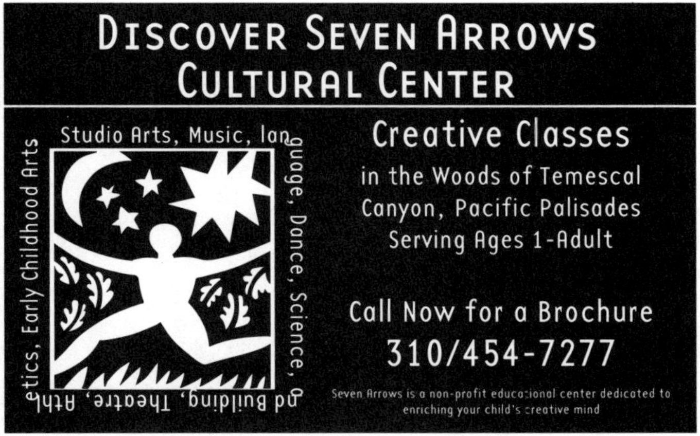

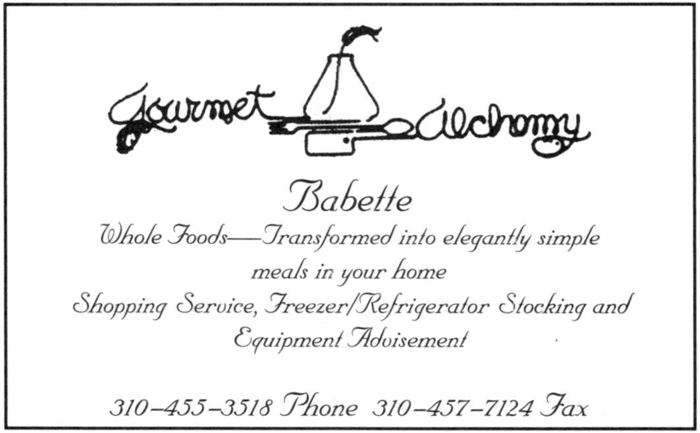

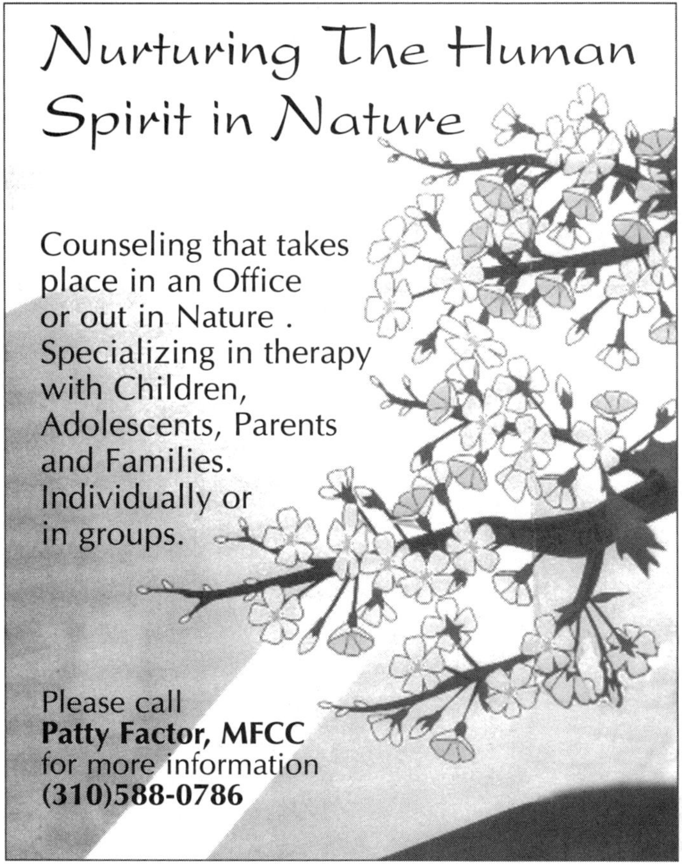

healing hands

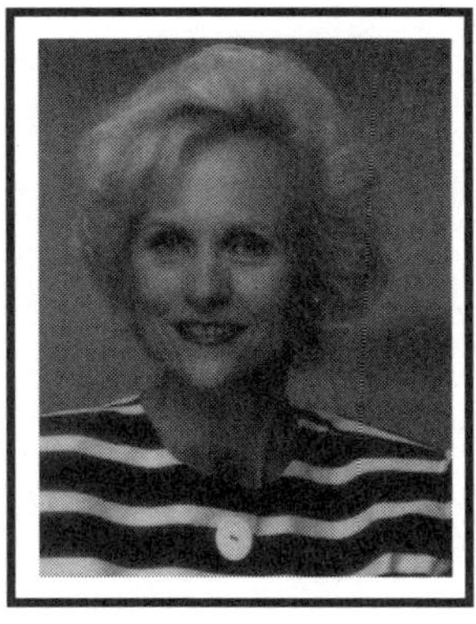

Zsuzsanna T. Krausz, C.M.T.
Reiki Master

Therapeutic Massage
Reiki Healing during Pregnancy
Reiki Healing Energy Sessions
Acupressure
Deep Tissue Release
Reflexology Foot Massage

Individual & Group Reiki Classes
1st & 2nd Degree

Mon.-Fri. 9:00am-7:00pm
Sat. 9:00am-2:00pm

310/373-9682 310/764-0436
South Bay Location

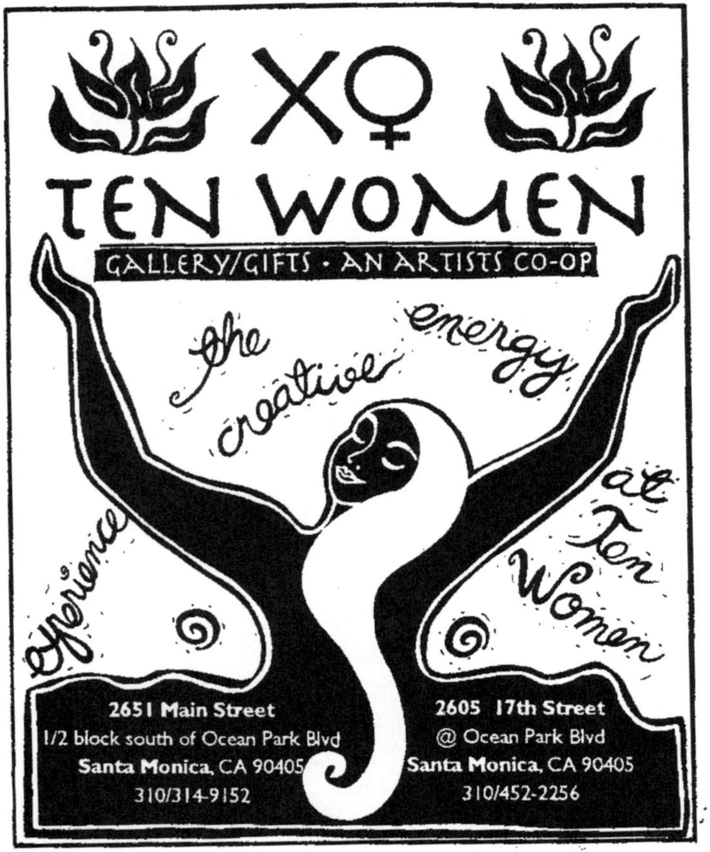

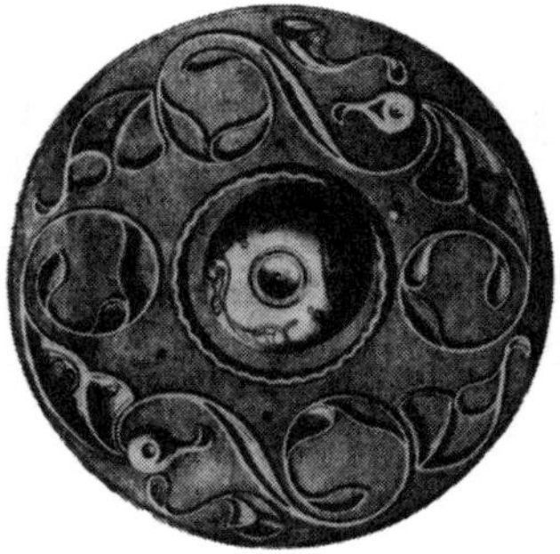

Barbara Shore, Ph.D.C.

Psychotherapy

1460 7th St., Ste. 306
Santa Monica, Ca 90405
310-208-3213

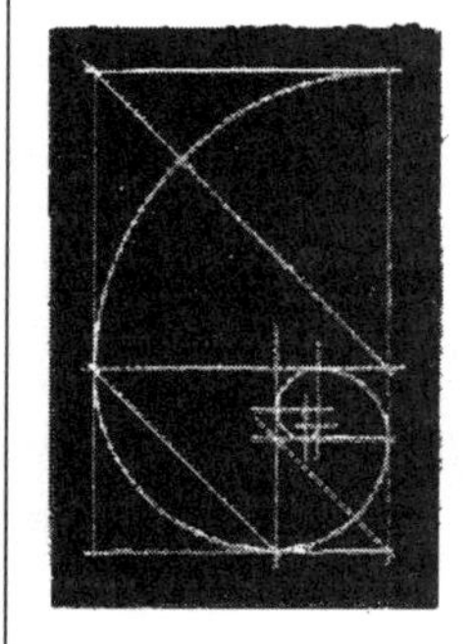

DURGIN CHIROPRACTIC

Pamela Sue Durgin, N.D., D.C.

Director of Naturopathic Medicine
Doctor of Chiropractic

612 Santa Monica Blvd.
Santa Monica, CA 90401
310.576.6176

Living Wellness

If you or anyone you know is interested in participating in next year's edition of "Living Wellness", please send us your name, address and telephone number at:

"Living Wellness"
21857 Koontz Way, Topanga, CA. 90290
or call 310-455-2714 for information
www.livingwellness.com

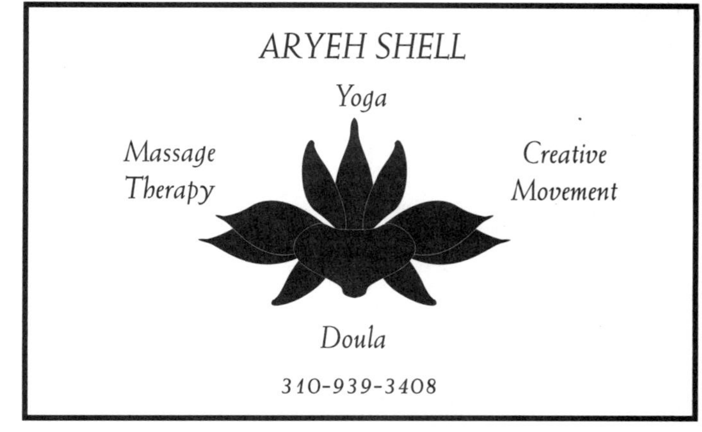

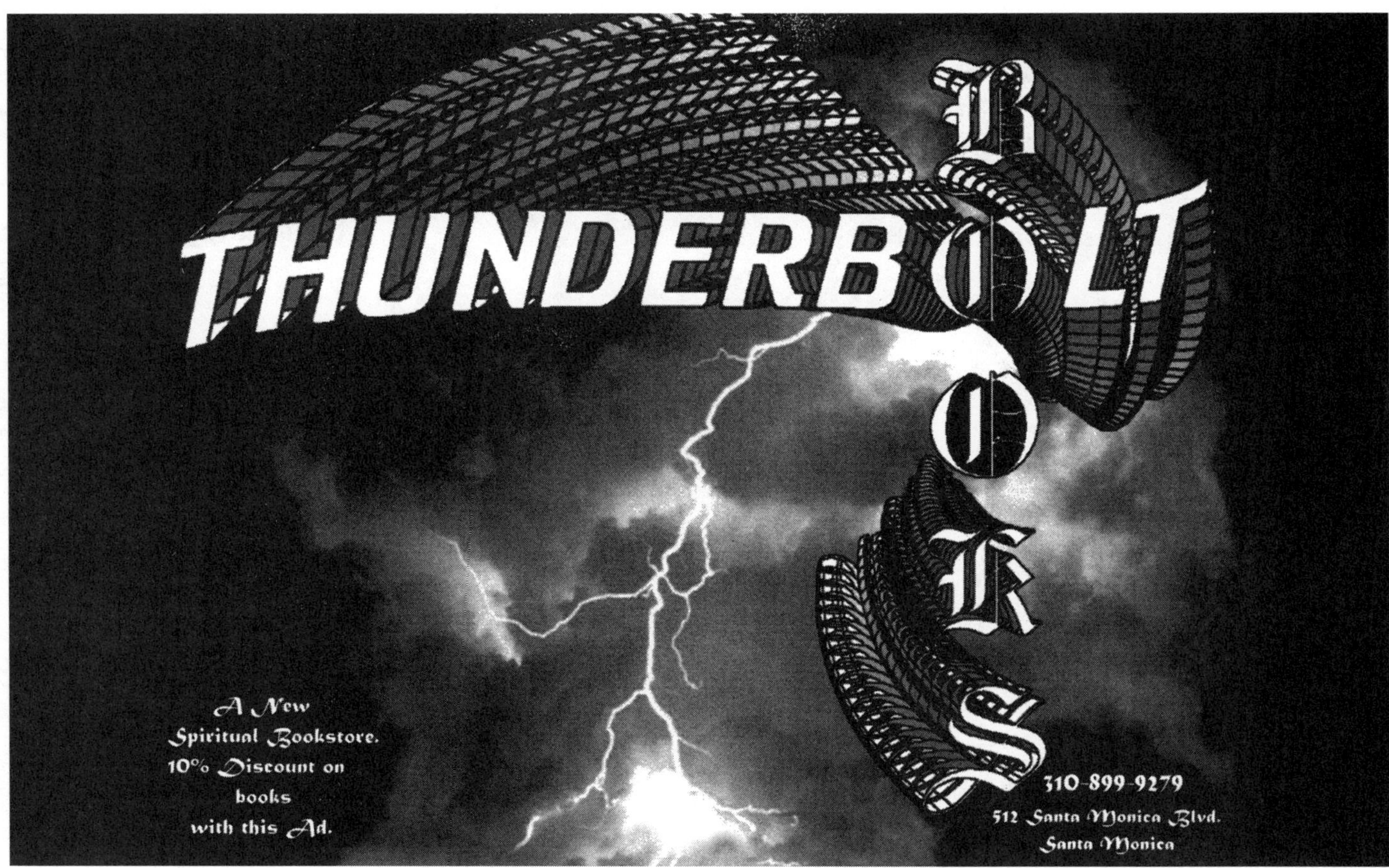
THUNDERBOLT BOOKS
A New
Spiritual Bookstore.
10% Discount on
books
with this Ad.
310-899-9279
512 Santa Monica Blvd.
Santa Monica

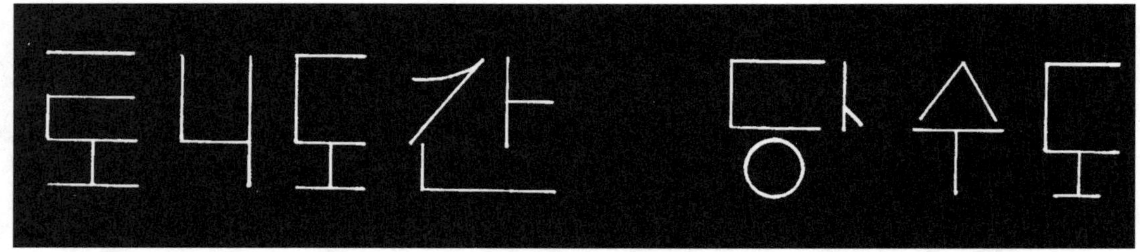

MONTGOMERY KARATE

"If there's no enemy within, the enemy without can do us no harm."
—African proverb

"There is nothing that I can do something about, if it's nothing but to adjust myself
to an unpleasant situation so that it doesn't destroy my spirit.
I am here to tell you that if you are seeking a goal, being
successful in reaching that goal will require all of the discipline that one can
muster from within their body."
— Napolean Hill

Children, Women and Men.
Topanga/Los Angeles

(310) 455-9557